YOUR BIOENERGY

YOUR DOCTOR

Fighting Illness with Energy

Tihomir Bralić

ATLANTIC

PUBLISHERS & DISTRIBUTORS (P) LTD

Published by

ATLANTIC

PUBLISHERS & DISTRIBUTORS (P) LTD

7/22, Ansari Road, Darya Ganj, New Delhi-110002
Phones : +91-11-40775252, 23273880, 23275880, 23280451
Fax : +91-11-23285873
Web : www.atlanticbooks.com
E-mail : orders@atlanticbooks.com

Branch Office
5, Nallathambi Street, Wallajah Road, Chennai-600002
Phones : +91-44-64611085, 32413319
E-mail : chennai@atlanticbooks.com

ISBN: 978-81-269-1883-6

Printed in India at Nice Printing Press, A-33/3A, Site-IV, Industrial Area, Sahibabad, Ghaziabad, U.P.

Space is an Inexhaustible Source of Energy;
Man is Part of the Space;
Man is—Energy!

Author's Disclaimer

This material has been created solely for educational purposes. The author and publisher are not engaged in providing medical advice or services. The author and publisher provide this information, and the reader accepts it, with the understanding that everything done or tried as a result from reading this book is at his or her own risk. The author and publisher shall have neither liability nor responsibility to any person or entity with respect to any loss, damage or injury caused, or alleged to be caused directly or indirectly by the information contained in this book.

Preface

In many years of my bioenergotherapeutic practice, treating a large number of diseases and conditions, I have achieved more than good results, which were, almost regularly, registered by (medical) doctors, when patients went to them for a check-up, after a certain number of my bioenergetic treatments.

I have no intention of putting the accent on my contribution in healing the patients, but foremost to offer the readers a series of advice by which the condition of their health will improve.

Believe me, it is possible, very much possible! By means of my optimism on the advice and the ways you can help yourself, which are described in this book.

Doctors help you in their way, medications help in their way, I help in my own way. Yet, everything can go much faster, and the effects of the treatment can be better by your own contribution and with the aid of the advice I am offering.

The stake is small, the gain is big, and therefore I am hoping that you will accept at least some of the advice offered in the text, and this text will hence justify its creation.

Tihomir Bralić

Contents

Demystification of Bioenergy

1

Many people baselessly attach the term "supernatural phenomenon" to bioenergy. In that sense, bioenergy is known to the general public, but since this natural phenomenon (not supernatural) is not yet sufficiently explored, it is being needlessly and baselessly mystified, especially in so-called "specialized magazines", which are allegedly dedicated to supernatural phenomena. Bioenergy is even often identified as magic, which is, mildly speaking, totally groundless!

Relying foremost on many years of my bioenergotherapeutic experience, I have come to certain solid conclusions in favor of demystification of the phenomenon called bioenergy. I will make an effort in giving several clarifications about it, so you wouldn't be deceived by baseless statements of individuals who have declared themselves great experts in this field. Some have, for instance, written that people with impaired health, who opt for bioenergetic treatment, and believe in that phenomenon, have a 50% bigger chance of healing than those who don't believe! That claim is utter nonsense, and here is why.

Patients have come to me who would, from the very start, tell me that they don't believe in bioenergy at all and that there is not the slightest chance that I could help them. I have never, nor do I intend to, tried to convince anyone in the need to believe in this natural phenomenon, because there is simply no reason for that. Moreover, that kind of believing or not believing is not worth mentioning. When I am treating someone, his/her psyche can "resist" all it wants; it will be to no avail, because during the treatment it is only the organism of the patient that counts. If the organism is damaged and in a bad energetic state, it will receive energy, whether the patient wants it or not. It is because this is a fully natural process, and in favor of demystification of this phenomenon, I will say only this: it is just a form of treatment, nothing else!

Word or term 'bioenergy' has it's origin in Greek word *bios* (life); therefore, in translation, this word means life energy!

That is the energy that activates, mobilizes, but also serves as protection of the organism. Every man has bioenergy, only it is in most people static, weaker, and in very few people it's stronger and mobile, which enables them to transfer it to other organisms. In the general public prevails the opinion that the bioenergotherapist "borrows", gives his energy to another, weakened, organism, which is wrong; he is a kind of a transformer, a transmitter of energy which is there, around us and in space!

I have already said that every man possesses bioenergy, some weaker, some stronger; I add that everyone can, through some exercises, in time increase the percentage of his/her bioenergy in organism, but more about that later.

Due to the decrease of bioenergy in human organism, there comes to a decrease of resistance of cells and organs to negative influences, which lowers their vitality and weakens the defense mechanism. There comes to a disruption of energetic balance of the organism and certain organs become exposed to risk of some illnesses. By recharging the organism with certain amount of energy (by one way or another), energetic balance is reestablished and the organs which have until then been threatened, can and do restore vitality and again perform their functions successfully.

In many books and articles in magazines, around the world, the authors deluge their readers with advice on nutrition and recipes with the application of which they could significantly improve their health, even completely heal from various illnesses. Nutrition is an important factor in life; still, I would like to point the attention to the appearing of, in aforementioned books and magazines, confusing bioenergy with the energy that the organism creates in itself by absorption of food and nutritious matters. That is mechanical energy which largely depends on the contents and quality of food consumed.

On the other hand, bioenergy resides in an organism, already existent, with a clear and formed identity. One cannot influence its creation in a mechanical way; it is an integral part of our being, unlike food.

It is important to point out that bioenergy can in no way harm the organism, which can't be said about food.

A certain percentage of bioenergy, although negligible, is contained in some kinds of food. By treating people with bioenergy for years, I have almost regularly noticed that obese people have, speaking in percentages, much lower level of bioenergy in their organisms, when compared to others. So the well-known saying that "Energy enters the body through the mouth" can be seriously questioned.

One factor of great importance for maintaining energetic balance, along with others, is breathing.

Breathing enables life, that is well-known. But few people know that the way in which we breathe can affect the quality of our lives, both in a positive and in a negative manner.

From the psychological point, uniform, even, especially breathing with the stomach, contributes to the feeling of being relaxed. That way, the organism is ready, has an important precondition for normal functioning, with a significantly reduced risk of biological disruptions.

Proper breathing also strengthens the defense against stress, which has, due to the increasingly fast tempo of living and growing number of situations that cause the disorders of the nervous system, become one of the biggest enemies of people's health, with immeasurable consequences.

We will later describe several ways in which you can improve the quality of your breathing.

Everyone knows that the sun is the source of life. It provides warmth selflessly to the 8,400,000 species of living beings (the number known to science), among them, of course, to human beings.

Man is not only a product of nature, he is a part of it, it can even be said that he is nature itself, and that all natural laws and manifestations happen in him. Therefore, everything that happens in nature happens also in a man, in an interdependent relation.

Bieoenergy (life energy) is a part of the total energy which surrounds us and which is being used by every life form on the planet. The acting of bioenergy is an especially important part of the natural processes that influence us. You may be surprised by the information that animals and plants also use bioenergy.... With the decrease of this kind of energy in them also, disruptions appear.

I have provided bioenergotherapeutic services, you may not believe, to animals (usually dogs), but also to plants, flowers, when they were "near death"!

I was visiting a friend once. We were chatting, when I noticed that his wife is taking a flowerpot with visibly faded pelargonium, intending to move it into a bigger box, which was supposed to end up in garbage soon. I have asked the hosts to postpone that and allow me to devote myself for ten minutes to the flowers—to borrow a wholesome dose of bioenergy to the faded pelargonium. Of course, they thought I was joking, but to my insistence they have agreed, smiling all the time and not concealing their disbelief. I have done my "treatment" in another room and the flowerpot was put back to its place. Tomorrow afternoon the wife of my friend called me on the phone. Notably excited, she informed me that the "miracle" has happened; the flowers were alive again, they have risen and recovered, avoiding a sad end—in a dumpster.

It wasn't a miracle, as the wife of my friend had said; simply, a plant is a living being which also needs energy to survive, bioenergy. The word "miracle" was also used by the owners of the dogs to whom I would occasionally give help, because most people are wrong, thinking that only a man is a living being that needs bioenergy to live.

We have already said that the Sun is the "source of life". If it wasn't for the Sun, there wouldn't be any life on the planet; therefore, energy of the Sun is precious for every living being. I am not exaggerating when I say that bioenergy is a pressing need of every organism! Any disturbance of its level in an organism, disturbs the process of cell reproduction and functioning of the organs in general, which then facilitates the emergence of illness. Luckily, there are ways in which the level of bioenergy can be held under control and hence eliminate the possibility of weakening an organism's defense mechanism.

Even in cases when illness has already "arrived" in some of the organs, it is possible to restore the temporarily lost quantity of precious bioenergy. Not only with the help of the bioenergotherapist, You yourself can contribute to restoring the energetic balance, which is an unavoidable condition for normal functioning of the organism, and that way help a "wounded" organism get back on track, at least in terms of a satisfactory percentage.

About this self-help and the ways it can become a precious ally of your organism you will be, in a more concrete manner, informed in some of the pages that follow.

I suppose that many of you have seen an event when a child hurts itself, for instance, by accidentally hitting a chair, table or something similar, or falls to the ground. In cases like that, it's usually some of child's limbs that is exposed to impact. Clearly, that is followed by pain in the injured spot and usually, with the cries and tears of the child. Almost regularly, a mother hurriedly approaches the child and says "Come here, mummy will kiss and it (the pain) will go away." Then she actually kisses the injured part of the body and most often the child stops crying, because the pain has indeed decreased or completely disappeared.

I have described this example in order to point to the fact that lips are one of the major transmitters of energy! To some it may seem naive or funny, but still, think about this: isn't it well-known from time immemorial that kissing with a partner is extremely pleasant to people and that it mainly causes pleasant flow in their bodies? That's a kind of "bioenergy exchange", and I'll leave to you the judgement on the accuracy of this claim.

Even the adults, when they receive a blow, say in the shoulder, elbow, or any other part of the body, spontaneously direct their hand toward the injured spot and keep it there for a certain period, depending on the strength of the blow and intensity of the pain that has appeared.

This reaction also can't be coincidental. Radiating energy from one's own hand evidently contributes to the easing of the pain. That is one more proof that bioenergy exists, that it is important and effective.

"Listening to the Organism" 2

You were at the doctor's and, after the examination, he/she has told you an unpleasant diagnosis. That stroke your self-confidence and fear has arrived.

In principle, that is a human, expected reaction, which still doesn't deserve that much importance, importance which can easily be transformed into additional psychic burden, which may further complicate the situation you are in.

The doctor has ordained a therapy for you, you have got your medications, and you are leaving the ordination with anxiety. There is no reason to worry, don't let it happen to you, keep your head up! Illness is an uninvited and unwanted guest, which should under no circumstances be underestimated, but one thing is for sure: no one is invincible, no matter what it's called.

Your doctor, who has spent so many years studying and fighting the enemy that has just "declared war" on you, is well armed with knowledge, but also with faith in the possibility of victory over it. If it wasn't so, he/she would not be doing the job he/she does, right?

Therefore, you already have one expert, strong, persistent and firm ally (the doctor), which is a good, optimistic sign in a battle that is ahead of you.

If you intend to hide your health problem from the members of your family and close friends, I advise you not to do that; it can be counterproductive, because when—sooner or later, they discover your secret (it usually happens), and find out that you haven't confided to them—they could interpret it as a sign of your mistrust in them. Some of them could be hurt and they could turn their backs to you in what is an unpleasant situation for you, and leave you, unnecessarily, without the valuable help of those who care about you.

Their closeness and optimism with which they would surround you would greatly contribute to the strengthening of your psychic stability and growing of hope in you, which is one of the more important preconditions on the road to victory of the organism over the illness.

Regarding the aforementioned, there is a need for another advice: if you have confided to some members of your family or to friends and if at any moment you feel even the slightest touch of pity, write them off and stay away from them in the future. That is because pity is worse, more dangerous and damaging to a person than all illnesses put together!

Regarding the illness against which you need to fight, try to think about it as rarely and briefly as possible, although it will in many ways try to occupy your attention, with intention to move you away from the normal life, making itself therefore "master of your destiny". You can't allow that, no way.

If you are mobile or at least limited mobile, use every chance to move, because salvation is in moving, not just lying in bed. When walking, do not look at your watch; as long as your organism allows you to move, do it freely, relaxed, do not worry—your organism will certainly "notify" you in time when you should rest.

So, you should "listen to your organism" and there won't be any problems.

Regarding food, I also advocate "listening to your organism". It is only logical that if you would eat something that doesn't make you feel good, you will soon give it up, because some of your organs would "protest". Occasionally, allow yourself the luxury of having the kind of food you would consider one of your favorite, but which has been forbidden for you to eat by your physician, due to the nature of your illness. Of course, this should be done moderately, in small quantities, just to satisfy your craving. My opinion is that this little "excursion", in spite of doctor's advice, can't harm you organically, while on the other hand it is very useful for your psyche. Naturally, this kind of "excursion" excludes taking fatty, so-called "heavy" foods, don't even think about that.

Burdening the organism with too fat food, especially in larger quantities, is known by many as "suicide from the plate"!

I also think that one should eat only when they feel the need for food, not according to some set schedule.

Every organism is a story for itself, every organism has its specific needs and habits that need to be respected so we wouldn't, knowingly or unknowingly, hurt its metabolism. I say that the needs of the organism need to be respected, but especially when it comes to food, moderation is essential in keeping one's good health.

If an illness hasn't caused weakness and exhaustion of your organism significantly, I dare recommend something that you most probably haven't done before: occasionally, e.g. once a week or once in a fortnight, do not take food for an entire day, but significantly increase the quantity of fluid intake on that day. In the evening, and hour or two before going to sleep, eat a piece of toast or a smaller piece of bread crust, if possible of a black bread. During the day, do not pay attention to the bowel howling. It is a kind of a shock for the bowels, but what is much more important is that this is a reliable way for an organism to "take a break", clean itself and get rid of large amount of negative substances—toxins. If you think that you are not in a condition that would allow you to fulfill these conditions for cleaning the organism and that it would be a risky adventure—I advise you not to try it after all.

In the following pages, there will be more suggestions for helping your organism recover, so if you have given up on the previous one, there will certainly be some that will seem less risky and easier for you to implement.

It is less known that fasting was conducted into religious rites with primary intention for a man to spiritually cleanse himself, as religious literature states. I agree that fasting, the deprivation of organism of food for some periods of time, affects the spirit—psyche of a person positively, that is evident. Still we must add that, starving an organism is (occasionally) useful in an organic sense also. That is a perfect opportunity for an organism to rest (especially digestive tract) from everyday, all-day, exhausting activity, with the duty to select the ingredients of taken food and make a decision on which to keep as useful to the organism, and which to discard.

Due to the increasing pollution of our planet, the question of quality of foodstuff we take into our organisms every day, and by that also the question of their usefulness or harmfulness, imposes itself.

Food is a source of energy that we all require. Although, when it comes to energy, I give the advantage to bioenergy, I will name a list of foodstuff I consider useful and some of those I consider harmful to the organism and which I personally avoid using.

The following food is prevalent in my menu:

Vegetables Salads
Fresh and dried fruit
Honey
Cereals
Plant fats and oil
Cheese
Milk
Eggs
Biological yeast...

I avoid, above all:

Delicatessen
Canned food in general
Meat with bigger amounts of fat...

Keep in mind that food, even the best food, if taken in large amounts, has a negative effect on the organism. Moreover, it turns into poison. Therefore, be careful, eat moderately, listen to your organism, do not put too much burden on it or expose it to unnecessary risks.

Most Tibetans start the day by drinking a glass of hot (not warm) water! This may come as a surprise to many. Let me clarify: Tibetans, whether they are ill or healthy, have done this for centuries. A glass of hot water taken on an empty stomach will certainly contribute to increasing the appropriate activity of digestive organs during the whole day! This may be repeated during the day, with the necessary precondition that water is taken on an empty stomach.

We do not need to talk about the importance of digestion of food for the organism, therefore I advise you to consider this kind of self-help a one-hundred-percent ally in achieving good health.

To this I may add that hot water also can act as a medication. I was present several times when someone suffering from gastritis or stomach ulcer, and doesn't have a medication on hand (usually Ranisan—based on ranitidine) complained about having strong stomach pain. My suggestion to them to drink a glass of hot water would initially cause disbelief and the thought I was joking, but they would usually listen and try. After approximately ten minutes, the pain would stop, to the surprise of the people present.

Reactions of the Organism

3

I would like to use the opportunity to point out the appearance of frivolous, or better said irresponsible behavior of some of my patients. I myself have perhaps contributed to such behavior by trying to achieve significant improvements of the health of a person I am treating already after the first or second session.

When I first meet a person that comes to me for help, I emphasize that it is highly desirable that we do five to seven treatment sessions. That is a number of therapies that in some way guarantees significant and visible improvements or even total healing of a patient.

However, depending on the kind of illness and its current phase, some of them feel so much better after one or two treatment sessions that they give up on coming to the rest of the agreed sessions. That is irresponsible behavior, because, simply said, we haven't finished the work we started, and I am not a wizard, in spite of what some of these patients obviously tend to think.

Some of them feel well even for a year, and then they call me in order to finish the treatments we have started.

Having that in mind, the doctors have a great advantage over me: they put a person in a hospital, keep him/her there for as long as they need, heel him/her, apply therapies and the patient is under their full control.

There are people who need a dozen treatments, when it comes to serious illnesses. The more an organism is damaged and endangered, naturally it needs longer treatment, greater quantity of bioenergetic "transfusion". Luckily, most of my patients honor the agreement on the needed number of sessions, so I am very satisfied to see them several years after, in good health and in good spirit.

There is a saying that any medicine that causes no reaction is not a good medicine.

I have already stated that the treated organism of a patient, later, itself selects the kind and quantity of received energy, which it allocates to the places where the causes of its problems are. If the problem is bigger in certain organs or body parts, those organs or parts require bigger quantities of precious energy.

Frequently, in such cases, an increased inflow of bioenergy to a certain organ or body part temporarily causes increased pain. Although I have pointed that possibility out to them, some patients forget the warning, the appearance of pain frightens them and they start thinking that their condition is getting worse, which is, as I have said, impossible. That is just a reaction of the organism to faster and increased acting of bioenergy, that is a fight of bioenergy against the illness, in which it is compelled to show that it is stronger, more powerful than the illness, while its manifestation may sometimes be an increase of pain.

Slightly more intense reactions of the patients happen (not with everyone) usually after the first treatment session. They are mostly manifested in increased flowing through the body, with occasional appearance of slight, bearable, pain, and only rarely in stronger pain. After every next therapy, as the health condition of the patient improves, the reactions are less intense, and soon they totally disappear.

Anyway, the improvement of the health of a patient can only go on an upward path. Because, I must underline again: Bioenergy cannot harm the organism, on the contrary!

A large number of people suffer from high blood pressure. Almost regularly, they tend to have dizziness, buzzing in their ears, limited head movements followed by "cracking" sounds when moving it sideways, up and down, their shoulders are visibly bent, they complain about the tingling of their hands, especially fingers, weakness in arms (they lose strength in them), pain in their shoulders....

With many of these people, pains are transferred to the lumbar part of the spine; sometimes they are stiff, the hips are also endangered, which causes sciatica, sometimes coxarthrosis of the hips; spasms of lower parts of legs are almost regular (especially at night).

That is quite of a list of problems, considering that the cause of all of them is at one place—ossificated neck part of the spine!

Bioenergy is certainly the most efficient, if not the only medicine that can successfully tackle the cause of the previously named health problems, neutralize and eliminate the ossification, and therefore remove, if not all, most of the hardships that appear due to the ossification of the neck part of the spine.

If you do not have "at hand" one of the good, tested successful bioenergotherapists, the exercise I have suggested for the spine, especially the one with "sticking" the fingertips in the neck part (that is a kind of bioenergetic self-massage), along with keeping your hands on the neck for 10-15 minutes each day can play an important preventive and corrective therapeutic role.

So, help is in your hands and your own bioenergy which, no matter in which percent it exists, can certainly ease your pains.

Take this seriously, because the spine is the pillar of the organism. Most health disorders tend to appear because of the endangerment of the spine by, most of all, fast tempo of living and great number of activities a person must conduct during the day, which require that the head be bent down for long periods, which ultimately leads to ossification.

Therefore, if you follow these advice, I am convinced they will be useful.

Alarming Pollution of the Environment

4

We have turned our backs to nature and have fallen into a trap we ourselves have set. During past several years, sudden and unpredictable climate changes are visible, which are negative in every way: ice on the North Pole is melting, heat and cold waves are interchanging almost over night, the mountains are moving, rivers are overflowing, more volcanoes are awakening, lightnings are striking horizontally.... It is all the fault of man and his decades-long pollution of the environment, with nature taking "revenge".

The calendar can, so to speak, only be of use as a decoration on the wall, and not as an orientation on the seasons of the year. Among other things, these changes have caused a sudden fall of immunity, weakened the defense mechanism of the human organism and it is getting harder to defend against rising number of illnesses and diseases.

With great concern, prominent doctors and experts from other fields of science, talk about the problem of pollution of the environment; they are warning, advising people to "come to their senses", that it is the last hour to do so, but unfortunately, with little effect. Pollutants care only about profit, while the statistics data on sudden rise of number of deaths on the entire Planet does not bother them, although they themselves, along with members of their families, are also paying the price because of their inconsideration.

Doctors have their hands full, they are doing everything within their powers to mitigate the dramatic situation, but it is difficult to fight a battle against the nature which is on the rampage, and we can freely say that illnesses have taken control over the world.

Near the end of the last century I have read in the papers a statement by a prominent French doctor, in which he had warned of the dangers of evident climate changes. He claimed that the pollution causes climate changes that are damaging for the immunity of the organism and, as I remember well, at the end he emphasizes that the only salvation is in connecting with bioenergetic flow, but that he doesn't know the way to achieve that!

Considering that bioenergy is "my field of expertise", I will try to help the reader to, as the French doctor said, connect with bioenergetic flows, with advice on the ways to achieve that. By that, the immunity of the organism is elevated to a higher level, a level that strengthens the defense system of the organism; at the same time, it is efficient in fighting health problems that are already present.

It will be a short course in bioenergy for the sake of self-help! Pollution of the environment is more and more evident, most of all, the pollution of air. Greatest burden is therefore on the lungs.

The lungs are the main part of the "breathing apparatus", an organ in which venal blood turns into arterial blood. We can say that they are the most endangered human organ, by the increasing number of polluters of the environment. Enemies of our health are numerous and dangerous, we shouldn't underestimate them.

Factories, especially chemical factories, emissions, broken chimneys, dust, polluted rivers, lakes, seas, etc. they are all "sources" of the pollution of the environment, pollution that strikes foremost at the lungs.

We who live in the cities are especially handicapped because we have very little time and possibilities to protect, at least to some extent, this important organ and refresh it by walking through the woods, or by the river, going to some of the mountains, and therefore finding shelter against the effect of the emissions we are all exposed to.

I have successfully fought with bioenergetic treatments against lung diseases such as bronchitis and pneumonia, with a large number of patients.

Regarding the problem of pollution of the environment, I have some simple advice that could be of some use.

The air humidity has also lately increased, which does damage to respiratory organs.

If meteorologists have pointed out increased humidity (although you can sometimes feel it yourself), close the windows. Open them when meteorologists notify you that the "danger" has past, or when you feel it yourself.

You should do the same also in cases when you feel that the wind is bringing unpleasant odors in the direction of your home. Also, in situations when you feel that the air outside is fresh and clear, use the opportunity to ventilate your home. Make a short draft, so the air would circulate through the whole apartment/house and therefore supply respiratory organs with precious help.

You are in the street as a pedestrian and you have stopped in front of the traffic light. Some of the vehicles near you are releasing emissions and you see that they are going in your direction. Before they arrive, react quickly: inhale deeply, hold the air in your lungs and move in the opposite direction from the polluter.

You should do the same when you approach the area of construction works, if they are causing clouds of dust, garbage lit on fire in containers, etc.

In such situations, it is important to react quickly, to determine the direction in which the air flow is carrying polluted air, so you would have enough time to avoid contact with it.

Thirst is Threatening the Planet

5

We have already pointed out that the climate on the entire Planet has changed in a negative manner. An especially dangerous problem for the human kind is almost daily drying up of wells and springs; drinking water is getting scarce, its quality is getting lower, that is a harsh truth, although the governments in entire world are hiding it from the public; under the pretext of avoiding spreading panic.

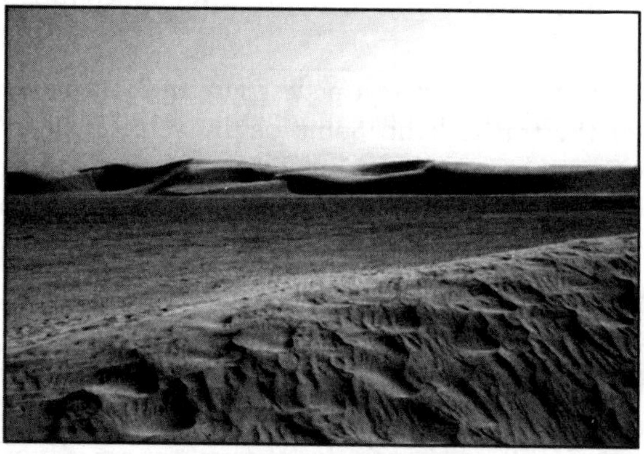

It is a known fact that a person can survive without food around forty days, while without drinking water he/she can survive at best four to five days. It is therefore not difficult to assess to which extent the biological survival of all living beings on the Planet is in danger.

My opinion is that we must urgently take action in order to protect the nature from further pollution, but that such action doesn't remain just on paper.

Every man can for himself significantly contribute to accelerating that action and making it more efficient by acting rationally regarding using that precious colorless fluid—drinking water. Otherwise, if we continue to act lavishly with water, a day when we will face an almost unsolvable problem, which can rock the balance of life on this already "tired" Planet is not far away.

Think about it well; it's not only about our lives, the lives of future generations are also at stake.

Radiation of Objects

6

Some time ago I have received a telephone call from an old friend with whom I haven't been in touch for a couple of months. He said that he had opened a boutique with exclusive clothes and shoes from Italy. During the conversation, he complained that business is not going that well, not nearly as good as he had hoped. I have sensed a tone of disappointment in his voice, but I have gladly accepted his call to visit him in his boutique.

The space was vast, and the look at the clothes on display left an impression that it really could be considered top quality.

We greeted each other cordially and as soon as we have started talking, a large painting on the wall, painted in oil, drew my attention. As soon as I looked at it, I have felt a radiation of negative energy, which has caused the sense of unpleasantness and unease.

I have told my friend that, to which he laughed, adding that he knows about my sense of humor, but that this one didn't succeed, although it had made him laugh.

I have waited for him to forget about the previous, as he thought, bad joke, and to take the far-fetched smile off his face. Then I told him, making sure he understands it's not a joke that all Objects Radiate, that they have their energy and that they, like humans, can spread around either positive or negative energy! I have added that in that way they influence the surrounding, and especially the more sensitive individuals.

He knew what my field of expertise is, but he didn't hide his disbelief. We have changed the subject of our conversation and he acted as he has been pleased by that fact. During our dialog, every time I looked at the mentioned painting it caused the same effects—increased feeling of unease, which intensity even increased, almost becoming unbearable.

My friend has noted that something is happening with me and asked me what was going on.

I have suggested that he takes the painting off the wall and puts it somewhere, for instance in a storage house or some other place, for at least a couple of days, assuring him that there are good reasons for that.

Whether because of our long friendship or out of curiosity, I don't know, he accepted my proposition.

He has called me a couple of days later. He was excited, he told me that a miracle has happened since he took the painting from the wall.

"Earlier, people have also entered the boutique, looked at the clothes on display, but rarely bought anything, so I was getting more worried by the day and more and more convinced that my decision to open a boutique was wrong. However, now most of the people enter the boutique, have a look, take the merchandise, pay and leave; unbelievable.... Is it possible that it has something to do with that painting?"—he asked.

I have answered affirmatively, to which he said:

"There is something in that, some devil."

I was bothered by the ending of his sentence, especially the word "devil".

"There certainly is something, but it is not the devil, as you have put it"—I reacted spontaneously.

I didn't try to convince him in the theory and the undeniable fact that all objects radiate; I assessed that it would be to no avail. I have no intention of convincing you either, everyone has the right to believe or not believe something and I respect that.

One of the factors which causes the decrease of percentage of bioenergy in an organism, which then causes the fall of immunity and "opens the path" to illnesses, is the pathogenic radiation to which we are exposed daily.

There are many kinds of negative radiation, but the biggest negative impacts are caused by the flowing of underground waters.

Dowsers usually practice discovering this kind of radiation, with the help of a pendulum or dowsing rods.

We are most exposed to the negative impact of underground waters radiation in the places where we are an “easy target”, usually those where we spend most of our time, if those are the places where this radiation occurs.

Damage from this radiation can be permanent, if a person is exposed to it for a longer periods of time, especially if it lasts for years.

Bed is the place where we spend most of the time, while we are sleeping.

We tend to spend a lot of time at home in general: at the table (when we eat, study, read, write, play cards, etc.), on the seat from where we watch TV, in front of the computer.... This also applies to the zone of the working desk at work.

According to the opinion of some of the experts that have conducted research in this field, geopathogenic radiation of underground waters, if a person is exposed to it, is damaging starting from 40% upwards. I don’t think this data needs any commentary.

I have already said that objects can radiate negative energy that is damaging for us. I am not quite convinced that I have succeeded in reducing the skepticism of my friend, the boutique owner, but I feel that I must try to do that with you; therefore, I will continue with this topic.

How can we avoid the negative impact of the radiation of objects that we are surrounded with?

Extremely sensitive persons feel an unexplainable hostility when in contact with certain objects, and, by inertia, they keep away from those objects. That is actually an emotional reaction of their organism by which resistance is manifested and these people, unconsciously, protect their organisms from an invisible danger.

If you do not belong to the group of persons that could be called extremely sensitive, with little effort you can enable your organism to be able to assess the quantity of energetic charge of certain objects, at least those that radiate very negative energy, and by that to avoid the danger to your organism.

It is desirable that you are alone in a room where there is complete silence. Try to think about an object that you consider especially dear. When you do that, if its size allows it, take that object in your hand and sit comfortably in a chair, or an armchair. Hold your hand in which you are holding the object close to you, little above the stomach, under the place where your ribs come together (where Solar Plexus is located). In comparison with emitting, transmitting bioenergy to another organism with hands, fingertips or the third eye, solar plexus is much more powerful and efficient. At the same time, it quickly senses even the weakest inflow of negative energy from the outside and reacts at once, by releasing a feeling of unpleasantness below the ribs and in the stomach. That is why I have advised you to put your favorite object on that part of the body.

Then take a deep breath, hold your breath for 7-8 seconds and then, slowly as you can, exhale all the air from your lungs. That is a relaxation breathing exercise. Repeat it 2-3 more times. When you feel that you are relaxed enough, try to "dive into yourself" and your feelings and ask your Myself how dear to you is the object with which you are exchanging energy by holding it in your hand. If the answer is pleasant warmness spreading through your body, inspiring positive thoughts, thinking about the bright side of life, then it is clear that the object deserves your affection and love and that it returns the feelings by emitting positive energy!

If the size of the object you consider one of your favorite doesn't allow you to hold it in your hand, put it on the table (or on the floor) in front of you, keep looking at it while doing the mentioned breathing exercise, make contact with it by your vision. It may take longer than with a smaller object, which is suitable for direct contact, but be sure that the "answer" will follow.

Repeat this procedure with the object that you usually avoid having contact. Almost certainly, it will stimulate the opposite feelings to those you have experienced in touch with your favorite object. Contact with that undesirable object will probably cause the feeling of emptiness, maybe restlessness, which will show you for certain that it's not a coincidence that you are avoiding it.

Negative Radiation of Underground Waters

7

We have already mentioned the negative impact of underground waters on our organism. Since this kind of radiation is the most dangerous for our health, I hope you won't mind me getting back to that problem which we could never, no matter how much we have addressed it, consider fully solved.

If you have never been in a church or a monastery, ask someone that has how they feel when they are in the Temple of God? Everyone, or at least a great majority, will tell you that they are overwhelmed by the feeling of bliss, total relaxation, while some of them may tell you that they feel occasional pleasant flows through the body.

Many of you will probably be surprised by this sudden "jump" to a topic of religious nature. I will explain right away: having no intention to belittle the contribution of faith in God by the people who visit temples and by clerics conducting rites in creating the mentioned feeling of bliss with the faithful, I must add that this kind of feeling appears also because of the known fact that monasteries and churches are never built on land that hasn't previously been checked for the presence of underground waters!

Examination of the ground is conducted by experts, dowsers, with the help of the pendulum, while in the past dowsing rods were used for this—this equipment is sometimes also used today.

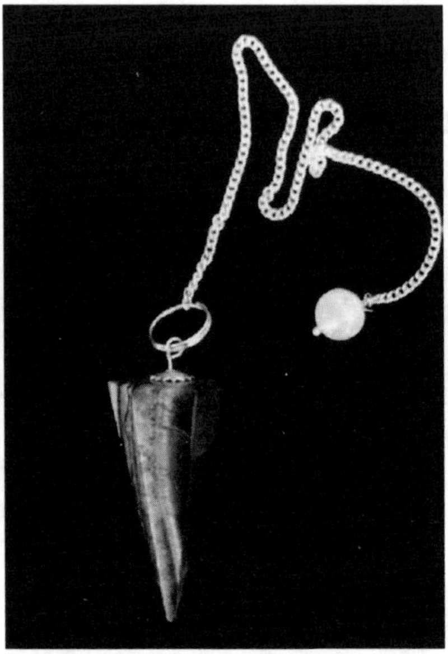

I have been informed from a reliable source that church has been practicing this for centuries, which undoubtedly proves that people have, since ancient times, known about the damaging influence of underground waters for human organism and that they knew that it is necessary to move to safety, to places that are out of range from this invisible enemy.

I have received a phone call once from a man who complained about his wife and him having, after moving into a new apartment a couple of months earlier, almost non-stop strong headaches, which are sometimes unbearable. He said that they have been taking pills in enormous quantities, but to no avail; they have been to the doctors, conducted "head to toe" examinations, even went to a seer, but the headache just wouldn't go away.

I have assumed that the causes of the problem were underground waters, so I suggested that they move the bed to other part of the room in which they are sleeping.

Two or three days later, the man called me and said that headaches have gone, both with him and his wife, and that they feel like reborn!

I don't practice dowsing professionally, I rely more on natural energetic "senses" and I gave those people the advice by intuition, which luckily had positive results. I have said this with intention to advise you how to act in a similar situation.

If you don't sleep well, if you are feeling exhausted, dejected, if some of the organs is bothering you, even though your physician has determined after examinations that everything seems to be in order, that is a certain sign that you are exposed to the impact of negative radiation of underground waters, probably during your sleep.

If you are faced with mentioned or other similar health problems, I advise you to move the bed in which you are sleeping into another part of the room, to a place that seems suitable and appropriate. Once you do that, after a couple of days—if the problems aren't gone—move the bed to another place again. Be persistent. Some of these new positions must turn out to be suitable, "healthy", because all the places in an apartment are almost never exposed to underground waters. That way, you will solve a big problem, without anyone's help and spare your organism from further trouble.

Our senses are, unlike those of the animals, imperfect. Therefore, if you keep a pet in your home, pay attention to the places where the animal likes to spend a lot of time, usually lying. It is almost certain that these places are out of reach of negative impact of underground waters; animals have a subtle sense and unmistakably feel that kind of danger.

You should try, at least for a couple of days, to "borrow" the favorite place of your pet; move your armchair or your bed to that place. You will quickly find out that you feel relaxed, comfortable, that you are full of enthusiasm and that, after a hard day at work, it takes very little time to regain your energy. Don't mind the "protests" of your pet about claiming its territory, because it will certainly find a new place for itself in your home that is also safe.

I have already mentioned the pendulum. It is mostly used by dowsers for finding underground waters. Pendulum can also be used as a diagnostic tool.

There was a period when pendulum was "fashionable". In some specialized magazines dealing with supernatural phenomena, some "experts" have claimed that with the help of a pendulum one can "contact the other world", even with the dead, if you move it in circular fashion above your head?!

Since the number of gullible people is much larger than the number of suspicious, many have rushed to buy this piece of equipment. Unfortunately, profit of the sellers was once again much more important than the health of the buyers.

When this became a mass phenomenon, in the early 1990s, I have tried to warn people publicly about the danger from using pendulum in this way, but in vain.

Pendulum sellers have earned well, but unfortunately, with many people, mostly young people, circling the pendulum above their heads has caused vicious vibrations that have damaged their brains! I have had the chance to meet some of them. They are alive, but their psyche is destroyed.

So, if you are not an expert, keep away from the pendulum!

The Spine—Exercises

8

Vertebral column consists of short bones, vertebrae, 33-34 of them. Vertebrae are divided into 7 neck (cervical) vertebrae, 12 chest (thoracic) vertebrae, 5 loin (lumbar) vertebrae, 5 sacral vertebrae and 4-5 coccygeal vertebrae (so-called tailbone).

The first 24 vertebrae are mobile against one another, while the last 9-10 vertebrae are grown together and they form two bones: Sacrum and coccyx. The openings of all vertebrae form the spinal channel.

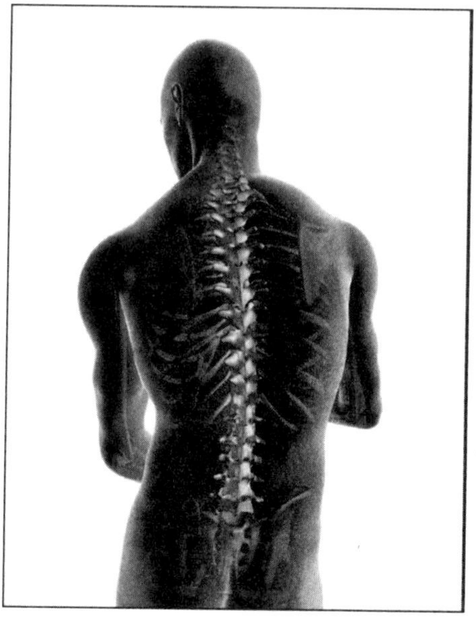

I believe that this elementary medical explanation of what spine consists of will help you better understand its importance and functioning.

Spine is the column of organism; it is an initiator of immense importance for the quality of living. Unfortunately, the spine is also affected by the increasingly fast tempo of living; it is under great pressure, without the time to "take a breather".

Therefore, almost every person has problems with the spine. Not so long ago, problems with the spine were usually diagnosed with the elderly. Today this rule does no longer apply. An increasing number of young people, including children, have problems with the spine, usually in the region of the neck, but also in the lumbar region.

Several years ago, conducting examinations in elementary schools in Belgrade (Serbia), physicians have discovered that an alarming 76% of the students have various problems and/or deformities of the spine!

I believe that some of the causes for spinal problems with children are: bags full of heavy books and notebooks that students carry on their backs, chairs and tables unadjusted to the age and stature of the students, but also small number of GYM classes. Those classes almost regularly consist of the following routine: one ball is given to the boys, one ball to the girls. Girls usually play dodgeball, while boys usually play soccer, and that is all. As for some athletic disciplines—not to mention gymnastic exercises—the kids haven't even heard of.

It must be added that the new generations largely contribute themselves to the physical weakness of their bodies with the passive way of living: they don't walk much, spend hours in front of computers and TV, sit in hunched position, they are prone to obesity. Most of them don't even think about occasional long walks or practicing sport.

I suppose that gym teachers in schools, having all this in mind, avoid working with children in a manner that would require better physical predispositions and readiness for greater efforts, in order to avoid children accidentally getting injured.

I have received a confirmation of this assumption from a school student from the neighborhood. He said to me that in his school, especially when they were doing some of the easier exercises on some gymnastic equipment (vault, uneven parallel bars or even on the floor), there were cases of students getting injured. He added that most of his classmates, both boys and girls, can't even do a somersault, which shows that young generations are getting less and less physically prepared for life. I think that this should be a cause for great concern and that the education authorities should respond to this, at least by increasing the number of gym classes in schools. As far as I know, the children have only two gym classes per week, which is not nearly enough.

In my bioenergotherapeutic practice I have many times registered spinal illnesses (mainly ossification of the neck region and scoliosis) at children of age 4-5! These findings have shocked their parents, because of the general belief that only the elderly face these problems.

Unfortunately, there are no more hard and fast rules regarding this issue. Almost everyone, regardless of age, faces problems with the spine, and that is an undeniable fact that we must accept.

While you are waiting for a bus, sitting in a restaurant or just walking, look carefully at passers-by. You will notice that great number of them is walking with visibly lowered shoulders, bent forward, with their heads bent forward; at many of them you will notice thickening in the neck region of the spine, limited mobility of the head left-right, that they are walking very slowly....

All these phenomena are caused by problems of the spinal column.

There is a long list of spinal illnesses, but most frequent are: Spondylosis, scoliosis, lumbago, discus hernia....

I believe that the biggest blame for the occurrence of these illnesses lies on the man himself! By the established "scenario", most people spend their days in the same way, which endangers the health. They get up in the morning, sit in the car, or a bus or a tram, whatever, then spend 8 hours or more at work, mostly sitting (there is also a question of having an adequate chair for proper posture), then they sit in the car again, go home, eat, lie down to rest or sit and watch TV, then comes bedtime, and they have hence practically spent an entire day with their bodies being very passive.

A great number of people are forced to sit with their head bent forward—when they read, write, type, at home or in the office, in front of the computer, in the car, etc. These actions usually last long, and that puts great demands on the spine, especially the neck part, which eventually leads to ossification, spondylosis. It can be considered a "professional illness", because the nature of the work these people are doing is such that it is necessary for them to bend their heads forward when working, and hence the occurrence of ossification of the neck part of the spine is practically unavoidable.

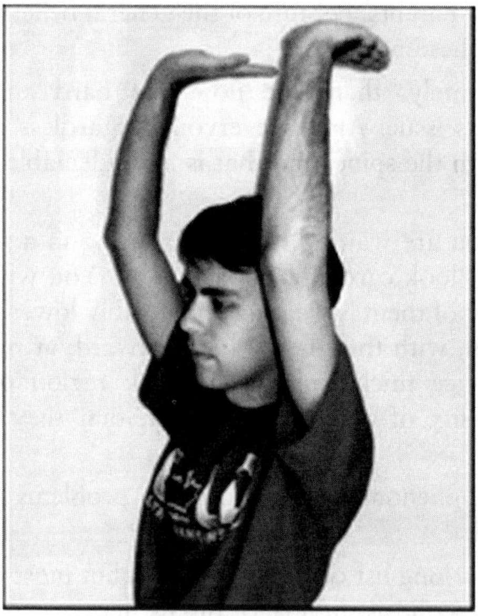

A man must work: study, write, type, drive a car, drive a truck, read, that is logical. Yet, there are ways to at least postpone, slow down and even avoid health problems caused by working, why not?

There are several exercises which I am certain you will find useful, especially for the spine.

1. When you are doing something that requires your head to be bent forward, if you feel discomfort in the way that you

feel as if someone has put an extra weight on your neck, if the situation allows, stand up, move away from the desk, raise your arms high above your head and keep them in that position for 2-3 minutes, then slowly lower them next to your body. Repeat the exercise several times.

2. If you are forced to sit, do the following: put the four fingers of each of your hands together (their tips), excluding the thumbs, put them along the edge of the spinal column in the neck part, press those parts hard with your fingertips and keep them in that position for a couple of minutes. Then stop pressing, but keep the fingers at the same place. After 2-3 minutes, increase the pressure again, also for a couple of minutes. Repeat all this several times.

Then put your hands on the table, and lay your arms, from the elbows to your hands on the table. Slowly move your head upwards. When you feel the strain, usually followed by pain in the neck, stop moving your head and hold it in that position until you feel that the strain and pain are gone. Then keep carefully moving your head upwards, again until eventually you feel the strain and pain. When and if that happens, keep your head in that position. When you feel it is safe, keep moving your head upwards again.... When you succeed in keeping your head in such position that your eyes are looking at the ceiling, the exercise is over. It would be advised that you repeat this exercise at least once more. By the same principle, you can do this exercise by moving your head downwards or left and right.

After this exercise you will feel relief, usually with increased clearness in your head.

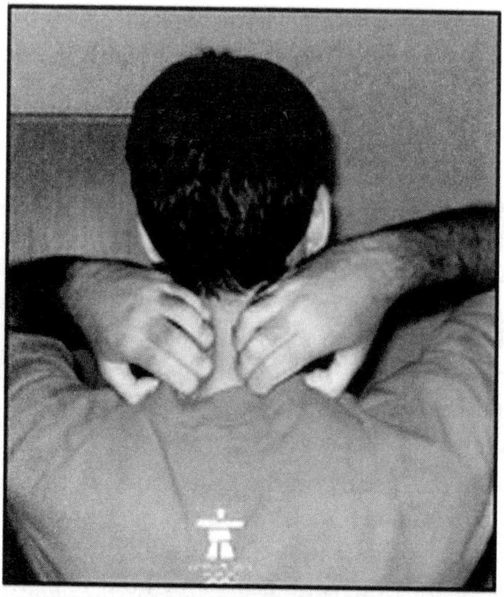

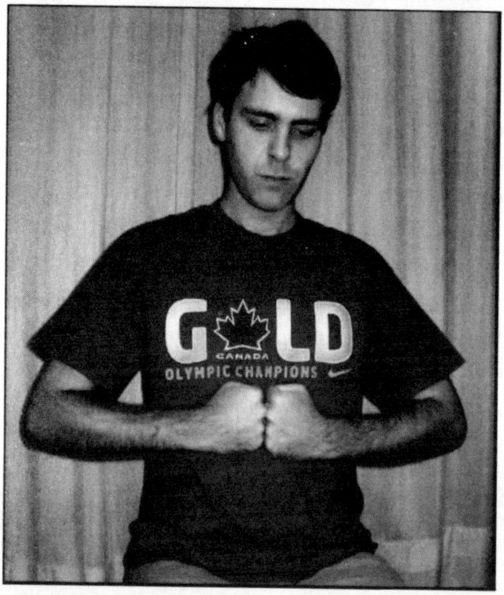

When you feel pain in the lower (lumbar) part of the spine, which usually happens after longer periods of sitting, you can help yourself by doing this exercise.

3. Tighten both your fists. Put the outer parts of your fingers together. Then press your fists against one another and keep the hold for 15-20 seconds. After that, stop pressing but keep the fists in the same position—together. Repeat this pressing routine for a couple of times and the pain in the lumbar part of the spine will significantly lessen, and very likely completely disappear.

One of the simplest and easiest exercises, which you can do in a chair where you are sitting, when you feel the tiredness of the spine is next.

4. Rest your whole back (including the shoulders) against the back of the seat. Put your hands on the lumbar (lower) part of the spine and stay in that position for a couple of minutes, while keeping your head as high as possible. The result of this exercise is certain to come.

For the next exercise a bed is used, but it is important that it isn't too soft, so that it wouldn't allow your body to change position by sinking of the mattress.

5. Lie down on your stomach with your legs stretched, put your arms next to your body with the palms of your hands facing the ceiling. Put your feet together and put them in a position in which the soles are facing the ceiling. Stay in that position for a couple of minutes. While not changing the position, try to raise and lower your head as much as possible in a consistent rhythm. Then slowly lower your legs in a stretched position and stay motionless for a few minutes. Repeat this exercise several times.

This exercise is useful not only for the spine, but also for circulation. I recommend the next exercise as important not only for the people with health problems, but also for the healthy individuals. You should also know that this exercise contributes to increase of the percentage of bioenergy in organism, increases its defense activity, relaxes and improves the circulation in the whole organism. I advise you to do this exercise especially after long periods of hard work—manual or intellectual, makes no difference!

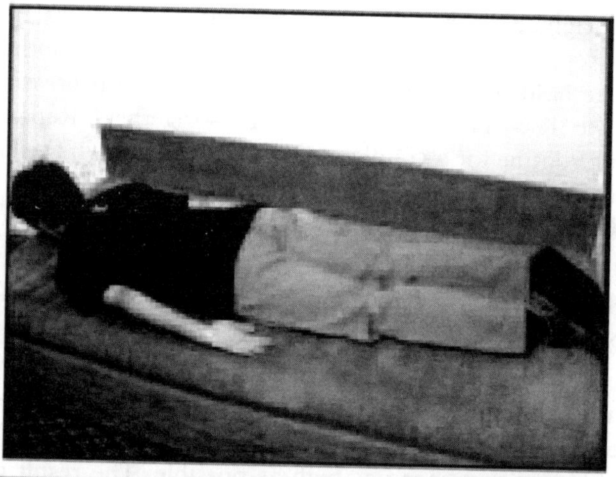

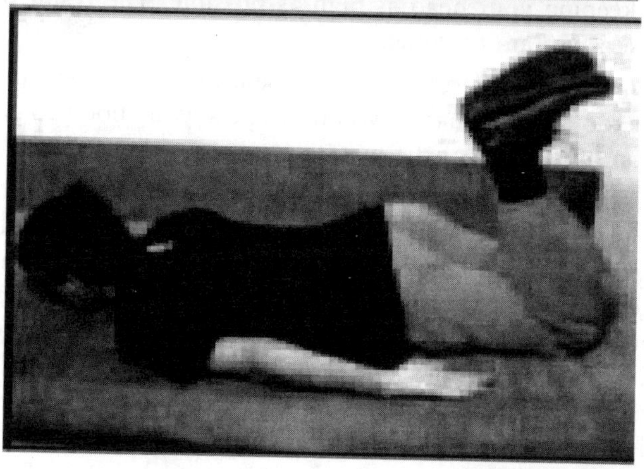

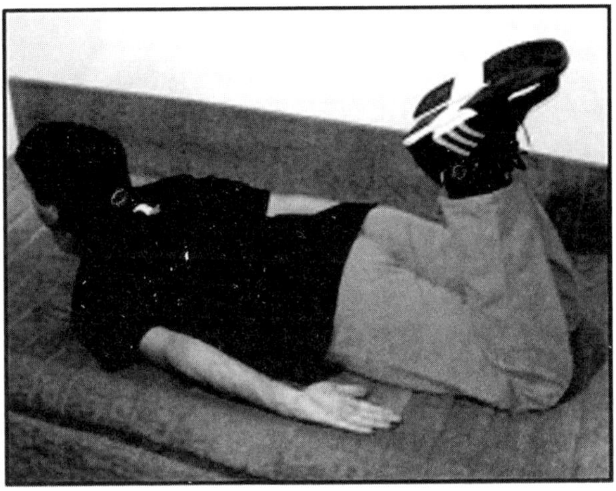

6. Stand with your arms loose beside your torso and your legs a little spread, not together. Raise one arm above your head (not too much) and put the palm of the hand horizontally, parallel to the ceiling. Remain in that position for 5-6 minutes, at most 10. After some time you will feel mild sense of "filling" the lowered arm with the feeling as if something heavy is flowing into it. That is due to increased inflow of blood. After the mentioned period, slowly lower the arm that you have been holding up. Look at both arms and you will notice that they are different in color: one will be rosy, while the other will be pale. Now raise the arm that you have previously been holding low, and leave the other arm lowered next to your torso. Remain in that position, too, for 5-6 minutes, at most 10. Switch your arms (up-down) several times. At the end, keep both your palms facing the ceiling of the room you are in, at least 15-20 centimeters from your torso, if you are able, for at least ten minutes. Then raise your arms, but this time with your palms facing your head. After 5-6 minutes in that position, the exercise is over.

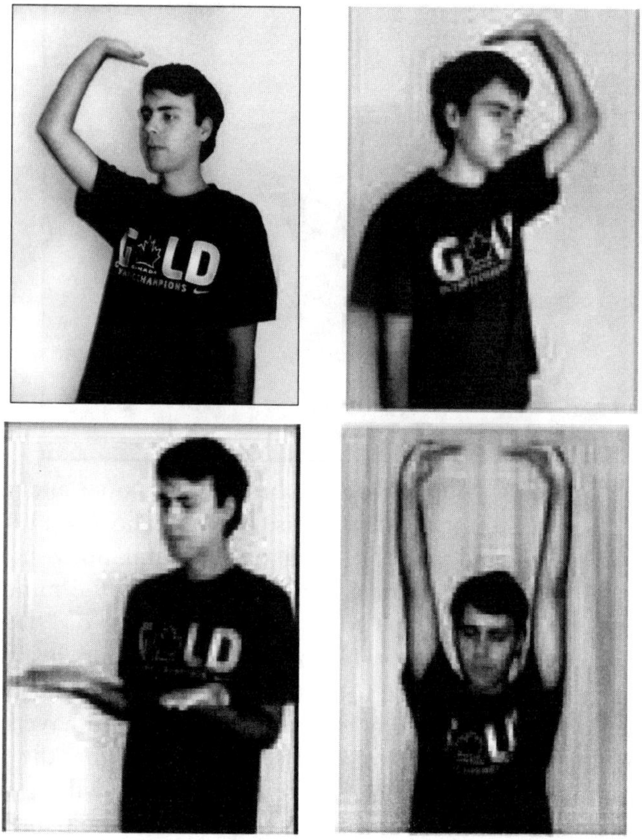

What follows is another exercise recommended for the people who, due to the nature of their work, spend most of the time sitting or standing.

7. Stand on your toes, so that your heels are 2-3 centimeters from the floor. Then abruptly lower your heels to the floor, when you will feel a slight blow and a slight shock to your body. The same thing happens during running and fast walking. Thanks to the vein valves, the blood will receive a stimulating impulse for moving upwards, towards the heart. The exercise should be done by lowering the heels to the floor at maximum once per second. Occasionally make a break.

A great number of these shocks would not be useful, because in that case, there wouldn't be enough blood between the vein valves and it wouldn't get to the veins. It is not recommended to cause more than 50 "shocks" by this exercise. It should be done in a fast manner, but not too fast, to avoid causing a headache. The shocks should be as strong as nature has intended, as during running. Therefore, this exercise is not dangerous for the spine or for the discuses. It is enough that you do this exercise 5-10 times, it won't fail to show results. The feeling of heavy head after long periods of intellectual work will disappear due to the impact of flowing of the vein blood from the head towards the heart.

I suppose that you have already seen or heard about someone having back numbness. It appears because of the vertebra springing out of position in lumbar part of the spine. The vertebra, therefore, presses the nerve and often doesn't allow the person even the slightest movement, because it would cause great pain.

This problem often appears when a person lifts heavier objects. Therefore, I believe that this preemptive advice will help you avoid the mentioned unpleasant experience.

8. When lifting heavier objects, try to be as close to the object as you can. That way you will use your muscles more when lifting, decreasing the percentage of participation of the spine in the effort, especially its lumbar part. You will spare the spine from being exposed to bigger risks, that could have grave consequences.

The bed on which you sleep is of great importance not only for the spine, but also for the quality of sleep. It is ideal if the mattress is not too hard, but also not too soft, in order to secure that your body is relaxed during sleep. Medium soft mattress prevents your body getting into unnatural positions during sleep, as well as unplanned premature waking up.

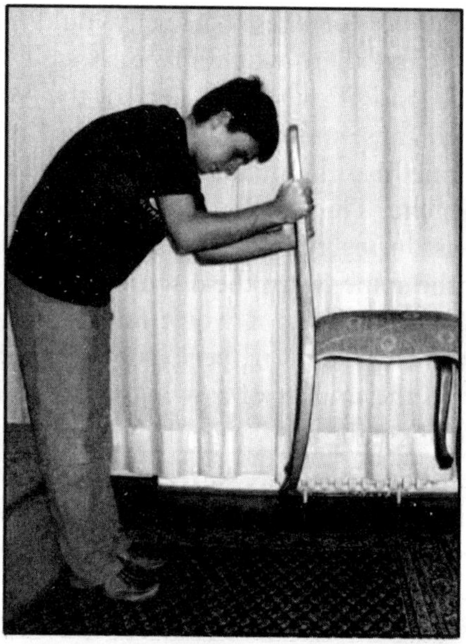

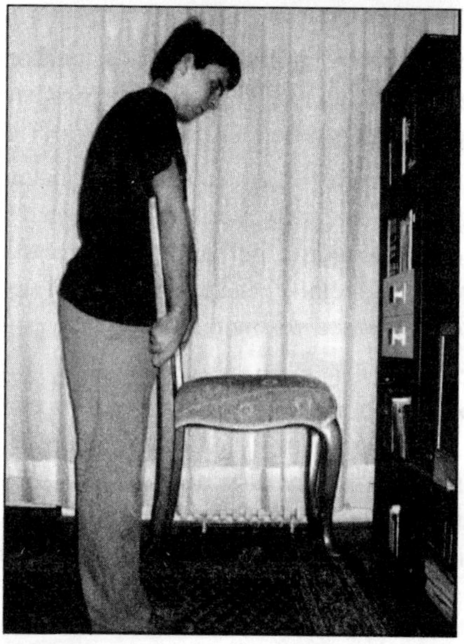

I recommend the pillow on which your head rests also to be medium soft, and what is very important—do not use massive, thicker pillows, which cause you to lie in an almost sitting position, in a period when your spine is supposed to be accumulating energy for the following day. Your spine may even be in strong pain in the morning.

It is quite often that people ask for help (usually the parents of children) in the form of back massage by stepping with bare feet down one's spinal column. Every massage is undeniably pleasant, but this kind carries a certain risk. An important precondition is that the "masseur" weighs no more than 50 kg. Also, he/she should be warned to advance slowly down the spinal column, upwards and downwards and to be careful to avoid his/her feet turning to the side, thus causing the vertebrae to spring out.

The Impact of Draft

9

There are different opinions about the effect of draft on our organisms. Yet, the majority believes that it is dangerous for health, especially the spine.

Most physicians believe people should keep away from draft. Several doctors I have collaborated with and discussed it didn't share the opinion of their colleagues. On the contrary, they had pointed out that draft is a natural phenomenon, which is not only harmless, but also useful for health. They have pointed out that quick inflow of air from the outside into the rooms where we spend time has a beneficial effect primarily on the lungs. I share this opinion.

I would like to add that this kind of impact on the organism can be considered useful only under the condition that it doesn't last longer than 15-20 minutes. I believe that longer exposure to draft can only be counterproductive.

I have recently treated a young man whose workplace is in a large factory hall in which he is exposed to constant, strong draft, which he can in no way avoid. Such is the nature of his work that he is "tied" to a place where he is exposed to draft practically all the time during working hours. He had a strong sinusitis and, as he had said, an unbearable headache in the forehead region, as well as occasional pain in his ears. He attributed those problems to the draft in his workplace, adding that he is close to a decision to quit his job and look for a job elsewhere, where his health would not be endangered. I have agreed that draft is the main cause of his health problems, considering the fact that he was exposed to it every day for many hours.

Draft can have a negative effect on the spine as well, even in situations when we are not exposed to it for a long time (e.g. several hours). That is especially true in summer, when the temperatures are high. If a man is sweating and his shirt is "glued" to his body (especially at the back, in the lumbar part of the spine), then he enjoys draft. But, he forgets that his shirt is in that way practically drying on him. After some period of draft, the sweaty shirt gets colder and its contact with the spine turns into danger. There often comes to stiffening of the back followed by pain, usually in the lower back.

Therefore, I believe that one should not take such risks and that it is desirable, especially in the situations when a person is sweating, to keep away from draft.

In the summer, draft is a danger for the spine while driving a car, especially on longer trips. Due to the high temperature, a driver is sweating. If the car isn't equipped with an air conditioning device, drivers usually open the car windows, and eventually there comes to a problem I have described—a welcome refreshment turns into a danger for health.

Therefore, an important advice to drivers:

During driving, if you are sweating a lot, stop the vehicle and change the shirt (try to have a couple of spare shirts in the car in the summer).

How to Defeat a Cold

10

A cold may not be what we would consider a dangerous illness, but it is certainly unpleasant. It lasts for several days and forces the person with a cold to avoid having contact with other people in order not to infect them. There can hardly be a person that has never experienced this problem.

Coming of a cold can be sensed in advance: runny nose, blurriness followed by appearance of tears in the eyes, feeling of weariness are clear signs that a cold "knocks on the door". According to the saying "better safe than sorry", you should react immediately to stop the appearance of this boring illness or at least shorten its duration. Put the palms of your hands on the back of the head next to your ears and keep them that way for a few minutes. Repeat that several times, and then put your palms on your chest, on your lungs. Hold them that way for ten minutes. You will feel the warmth transferring from your hands to your lungs. After that, return to holding your hands on the back of your head, then to the lungs again. Do this several times during the day, depending on how much time you have and the results will come. If nothing else, a cold will not last as long as it would otherwise, and it won't be as strong. This way of transmitting heat energy to the lungs also protects you from the flu.

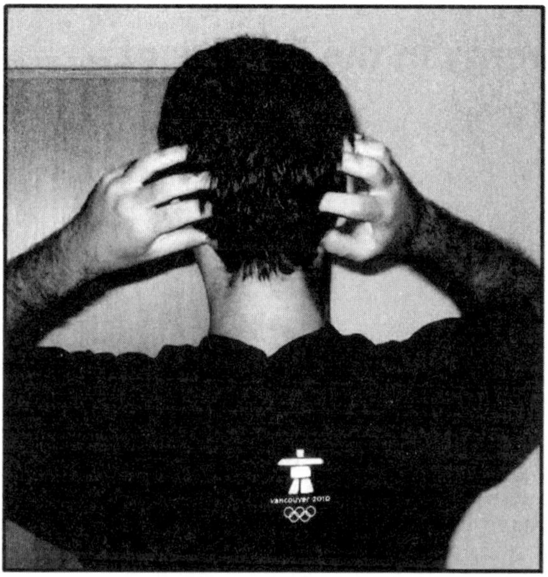

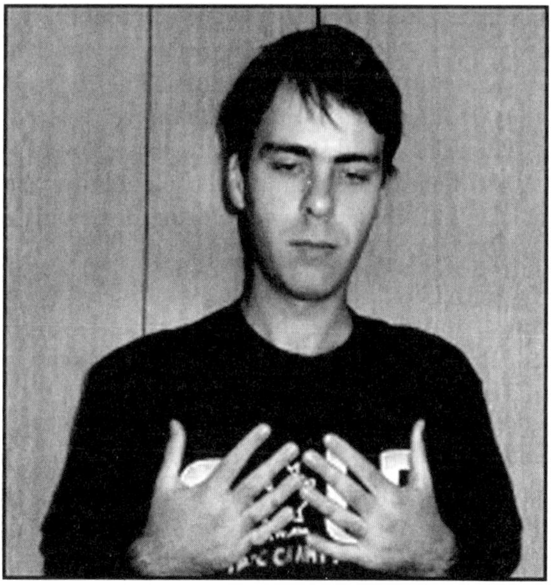

Another advice: during the cold, avoid using dairy products, cereals and juices; take a lot of natural vitamin C (fruits).

Bioenergy in the Service of Sport

11

A great number of professional athletes, mostly soccer players, have come to me for help. I have registered a problem with the spine of almost each one of them. I wasn't particularly surprised by that, because the spinal column of athletes is exposed daily to great strains at trainings and games.... Many of them have had bad circulation, which was one of the main causes of their frequent injuries.

I firmly believe that, because I have come to this conclusion by helping athletes. After a few bioenergetic treatments, athletes with poor circulation usually wouldn't come to me anymore, because they wouldn't get injured anymore, at least not that seriously. When they would get injured, and it would usually be a mechanical injury, due to improved circulation they would recover quickly and therefore wouldn't need to come to me for help.

The same rule applies to athletes who have problems with their spines. Injury-prone football players—after a few bioenergetic treatments, when their problems with the spine were solved and the spine would get strong enough to perform its role as the pillar of organism, fully prepared for the greatest demands—they would go back to the field. Maybe it will seem as an exaggeration, but since bioenergy has a stimulating effect, they would also play better than before! I have watched some games and seen it myself.

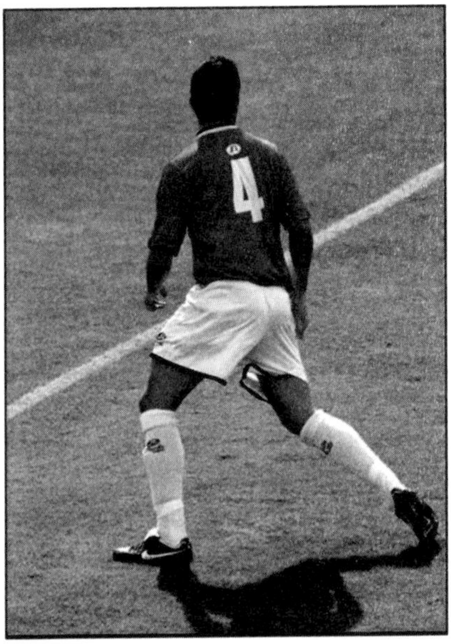

Several years ago, a football club from Belgrade, national champion at the time, had three players with difficult injuries just three days before the match against the famous "Bayern Munich". The public didn't even give them the theoretical chance to appear and play the game. The then president of the club has accepted with great faith my bioenergetic treatment of the players, with the aim to contribute to their quick recovery. To everyone's surprise, all three of them played against "Bayern", and they played very good.

In the same period, a well known football player (N. Bjekovic) of a big domestic club had a difficult injury. Since it was a difficult injury of the interior ligaments of the knee and since I have in the first contact established with him that he also has problems with circulation, the spine, ankle joints (he had confirmed my assumption), I have suggested to him that we do five treatments in five consecutive days.

Five or six days after the fifth treatment, he had started to train, to the satisfaction of everyone. It is especially important to emphasize, and that is the reason I have mentioned this player, that he has never had a serious injury after that.

One of the best players of a well-known European basketball club has injured his ankle joint in training, just two days before a decisive match. Keeping ice on it didn't help him and the club's doctor had told the coach not to count on him. A young athlete's friend drove him to me. Thanks to bioenergy, he has not only played, but was man of the match.

I repeat that bioenergy has a preemptive and a very stimulating effect on athletes; I am free to call it a natural doping!

At one time, a Romanian high-jumper, until then totally unknown to the public outside Romania, took with him his bioenergotherapist to European Championship that was held in Italy. He has won a silver medal, to the shock of the public, with the same height jumped over as the winner, but from more attempts! No one can convince me that the decisive role in this unexpected success hasn't been played by bioenergy and its stimulating effects.

Cooperation with Medicine 12

One evening I had a visit from an old patient of mine. He was accompanied by his twenty-year-old son, who was limping, dragging his left leg. When the boy sat in a chair, he lifted his trousers and showed me a big hematoma on his ankle joint. His father said that the boy is supposed to have leg surgery in the morning and that he has brought him to me to try to at least reduce the swelling a little.

After the treatment, the swelling has visibly shrunk and the father and son have left. Two days later, father of the boy called me on the phone. He said that the operation was successful. He added that the surgeon-orthopedist which operated on his son has said after the operation that he has never done an easier surgery, of the thousands he has performed: there was almost no resistance from the organism. My old patient had also said that he had revealed to the surgeon that we have performed a bioenergetic treatment prior to the operation with which we have reduced the hematoma. He just shrugged his shoulders and said: "Together we are stronger!" He didn't mind this kind of invisible cooperation of medicine and bioenergy, and I was very pleased because of that.

Since I have mentioned surgery (which I hold in high esteem), I will use the opportunity to boast about helping an excellent cardio-surgeon three years ago, whose hands were affected by arthritis. Illness was threatening to send him to early retirement, but luckily, it didn't come to that. He still does his job successfully today, and the fact that I have contributed to that fills me with joy.

I have already mentioned that during the treatment I feel in my palms how the organism draws one out of three kinds of energy (heat, electrical, magnetic), which allows me to diagnose a problem during the treatment.

Organism cannot "lie", it reveals its weak spots to me and therefore facilitates the therapy.

I have often pointed to the patients that his/her organ signalizes a problem, but then they deny it, saying that he/she has been to the doctor's just a month or two ago. The same case was with a younger woman with kidney sand that I have treated.

A couple of days later, I have met a neighbor, who told me that she has sent the young woman to me. After the treatment the young woman dropped by my neighbor and told her that I have pointed to her the problem with the kidney. "I'll go and visit my doctor again"—she said.

The examination proved me right.

There are many other examples of cooperation of medicine and bioenergy in the service of health.

Music and Energy

13

Everything has its energy—positive, less positive, neutral energy (children), negative, and everyone transmits energy.

Musical pieces and music in general are also a source of energy that affects the surroundings. I suppose that some of you may have heard about the experiments with playing various kinds of music and its effect on flowers. It was established that plants grow and bloom significantly faster with classical music being played than with rock, pop or jazz music.

The scientists have concluded that this is due to classical music being full of harmonious, relaxing tonalities, without electronic aggressiveness of the other musical genres.

Their conclusion is correct, but one can also say—incomplete?

It is less known that in the mystical East, especially in India, there is a so-called "om music". That is a group of tonalities, energetically perfectly harmonious with positive effect on the listeners, tones that blend into a melody on an energetic basis, in a way known to the authors from the East. I have had the chance to listen to that combination of tones and, believe me, I have never felt such relaxation and the tide of positive thoughts in me.

How important the sound, tone and its energy are is illustrated also by the following example that at first sight may not have that much to do with our subject.

As everyone knows, the car industry is in constant competition for a place in the world market and the engineers of all manufacturers are making great efforts in order to perfect their engines, with the aim to beat the competition. This shouldn't be understood as a commercial, but I have found out from reliable sources that working of the engine of BMW cars has a positive effect on the driver! That has been confirmed by several people who own a BMW. They clearly hadn't tried to determine the cause of it, but they say that, apart from calmness during driving, occasionally they feel that the working of the engine improves their concentration.

I have also found out from reliable sources that the experts from BMW have worked on the engine sound, making it to the model of om music! It may be so, but I'll leave a question mark to this claim?

Anyhow, energy is all around us, we are all energy and if we manage to control it and direct it properly, the results should be good.

People who are aware of the influence of so-called OM tonalities on a person mainly recommend listening to the musical works of one of the greatest composers, Wolfgang Amadeus Mozart. His works are said to be closest to the mentioned tonalities and have a positive effect on the listener. Just like the great scientist Nikola Tesla, they say that Mozart has been "colluding", being on a direct link with Cosmos and its energies, which has contributed to the grandiosity of his work. They corroborate this assumption with the alleged fact that the great composer never made copies of his works, didn't make corrections, never erased or changed a note, which leads to the thought that he wrote as if someone had dictated music to him.

I wouldn't try to confirm one or the other assumption. But it is a fact that Mozart is one of the greatest composers in history, an author of works of wonderful tones which transmit a perfect energetic harmony.

Energy: Cure and Food

14

In late 2003, people around the world had the chance to see a "wonder" on TV: a seventy-year-old man from India who hasn't eaten anything in 60 years! He is alive, and what is very interesting, in good health, which has been confirmed by an international team of doctors who have examined him.

The public was shocked and everyone wondered: how is that possible? Clearly, a great number of people have doubted the authenticity of the story, claiming it is some kind of a trick. Although the scientists, who generally doubt everything that can't be seen and touched, have confirmed that the man lives without food for so many years, many people still didn't believe something like that was possible.

Science says that a man can live at most 40-45 days without food. Logical question is then how could this man survive more than half a century, not even feeling hunger? There is an explanation for that: this Indian practices YOGA, which consists of exercise and meditation with the aim to be able to fully control his senses, which he has obviously achieved.

Another question which arises is how is his organism fed? The answer is: it feeds with ENERGY, cosmic energy that he manages to, with the help of yoga and meditation, transport into his body, therefore eliminating the need for food.

As human kind is generally ready to immediately cast away anything that goes beyond the established "scientifically determined natural laws", and that applies to the phenomena which people can't understand and explain, many people have thought and said that the mentioned Indian eats secretly, while just wanting to attract attention. Why would he wait 60 years, and in the age of 70 decide to "attract attention?"—I wonder.

Many have reacted in the same way to the demonstration of telekinesis (moving of objects just by looking at them), not to mention the YOGIS who walk on the water surface, which defies the known laws of gravity. There are also a great number of scientists who have disputed such "demonstrations of unnatural" because their work, as they say, is based on solid hard evidence, which can't be applied in demonstrations like these, so they are declared a deception?

Regarding that, the following question arises: if our sight registers a phenomenon, by our criteria inexplicable, does it mean that it doesn't exist? Should we treat it like we haven't noticed it? My opinion is: Not at all. Human knowledge is just a drop of water in an ocean: people must always be prepared to learn.

Regarding tangibility of evidence, on which the scientists insist, let's take for example the great scientist Nikola Tesla. His inventions have undeniably brought great benefits to mankind. Electricity, the impulses travel from one country to another, from one continent to another, although they can't be seen. Does that mean Tesla was a charlatan? Experts on his work claim that he has, during his entire life, been able to transfer findings into knowledge with ease because he had understood the secret of the eternal Space, that Space is an inexhaustible source of energy. He has focused his efforts to finding a way to transfer that energy to our planet and enable us to use it. Luckily, he has succeeded.

Not many people know that Nikola Tesla was an expert in yoga! He has practiced exercises "yoga hidre" during which the practitioner appears to be asleep, while his consciousness is fully active. In that state, the conscious and the subconscious in a person spontaneously come into touch. One hour of yoga hidre exercise is equivalent of about four hours of sleep. Tesla usually slept for 2-3 hours, never longer!

"I know how to fully immerse into sleep and therefore a few hours a day is enough for me to fully recover from psycho-physical efforts"—he used to say.

Did you know that Tesla avoided shaking hands with other people? He has had awkward moments because of that, but he didn't give it up. He was actually avoiding the possible transfers of negative energy from someone he shakes hands with. So, Tesla wasn't "weird", an exhibitionist, as some have labeled him, but a genius expert on energy and the ways of its transmission.

Bioenergotherapist also "borrows" cosmic energy and transfers it into an organism which, due to lack of energy, has health problems. Of course, it is difficult, maybe even impossible to explain the way it is done to "unbelieving Thomas's". Therefore, many people doubt the efficiency of bioenergetic treatments. Some even consider it a kind of "magic", which is ludicrous.

I have many times treated people with heavy medical conditions, in times when medicine had already given up on them. They have come to me usually without hope and suspicious. After a couple of treatments, when their condition would start to improve, which was confirmed by medical findings, they would usually say: "Thank God, a miracle has happened!" They went away in good health, believing that a miracle has happened, not leaving the possibility that it was in fact due to invisible and intangible bioenergy.

Of course I wouldn't try to explain to them how we have achieved the wanted result; it would only be a waste of time. The only thing that is important to me is that the treatment has a positive result!

Cure is All Around Us

15

Many of you have probably seen when a child, playing in the nature, sees dry chicken excrement, lifts it from the ground and—eats it! Also, some children sometimes pick their noses and then, with pleasure, eat the contents they have picked from the nose! It is not rare that a child also eats a crust it has removed from its arm.

A substantial number of not only children but also adults occasionally eat a piece of mortar from the wall. They all do it spontaneously, unconsciously, because they are simply "listening" to their organism that has signalled the need for these kinds of food, which many would deem unacceptable. It is not a coincidence. The organism knows, feels that these unusual "meals" contain ingredients that it necessarily needs, at least in some periods.

Therefore, if you see children or adults taking these kinds of "food", I urge you not to deter them; honor their cooperation with nature and their agreement with their own organism.

I suppose that many of the readers would deem shocking that a certain number of people have cured themselves from serious, even the most serious illnesses (cancer) by drinking children's urine! I have personally met some of them. Their healing has been confirmed by doctors that have previously set the almost hopeless diagnosis.

I didn't mention this with intent to advise you to heal yourself in that way, but with the intention to underline the fact, disputed by many, that we know very little about our organism, and even less about the ways an organism can be cured.

The Power and Ineffectiveness of Prophylaxis

16

The number of women with uterus myoma is lately on a dramatic rise. The doctors have warned about that through media, adding that women themselves are "to blame", because they don't go to regular check-ups, so medicine is unable to react preemptively.

I believe this claim to be unfounded, and here is why: a woman comes to the doctor's for a check-up and everything turns out all right. She comes again after 2-3 months, and again everything is ok. She comes to the doctor's next time—there is uterus myoma. So, I ask a question: how would that prophylaxis of medicine work? In which way could it prevent the appearance of the myoma at a woman who has regularly come to check-ups?

Medicine usually reacts and acts in a moment when the illness is already present. Therefore, speaking publicly about the "blame" of women for the appearance of myoma is, mildly speaking, distasteful.

My experience shows that bioenergy provides certain preemptive protection, halts the progress of the illness and, luckily, succeeds in defeating it in most cases.

Bioenergy is hence proven and reliable preemptive protection of the organism, while medicine usually treats the consequences. Bioenergy deals with the cause of the health problem. Yet, I wouldn't want this to be understood as contempt for medicine and its indisputable achievements in helping people. It has its place and no one can deny it, but everyone does what they can to help and every help is welcome.

Method of Work, Cases from Practice

17

In the early 1990s bioenergotherapy was modern. Many have practiced it, or better said, cheated and mocked people and charged it a lot. It's no wonder that official medicine is still skeptical about this kind of treatment. The fraudsters who were "practicing bioenergy" have contributed to that. Their "treatment" usually lasts for 2-3 minutes (not enough) and is often followed by religious preaching. When they have more patients, they do "group treatments"—even for thirty people at once, in order to finish as soon as possible. A woman had told me once about her visit to the "bioenergotherapist"—he has emphasized that it is important that she strips and stays only in her underwear. "In twenty years marriage, my husband hasn't touched me so much as he has in these ten minutes"—she had complained.

But every fashion comes and goes away, and so has this one. Today there are few people who practice bioenergy, who are serious and qualified. Since energy is a serious matter, it is not recommended to toy with it, especially with bioenergy, since it can become a boomerang with grave consequences. A great number of "bioenergotherapists" has stopped practicing it, due to force majeure. I have seen some of them and have noticed their evident mental problems, but also other health problems (boomerang effect at display). They are visibly "absent", some of them noticeably shaking, have difficulties moving.... Some of them have had terrible family tragedies, some of them have died. One of my friends often says: You can't build your happiness on the misery of others and avoid the punishment from above.

I share this opinion and add: bioenergy is certainly useful, but by practicing it in a wrong way, it becomes very dangerous for a person which out of ignorance, greed or something else exposes himself to unnecessary and grave risk.

Besides following these rules, which are the main prerequisite for successful practicing of bioenergy, energetic power of emission of the therapist is of great importance. Most people think that this is decisive, even the only important thing, but that is wrong. Only 0.1% of the bioenergotherapists reach the highest level of emission, so-called genetic potential—a level of emission that never weakens, as long as the therapist lives!

Many of my patients, which have previously visited another person for treatment, have told me that the "therapist" had, right after the beginning of the treatment, fainted—so they ran away in fear. The cause of that is mainly a minimal, insufficient power of emission of the so-called therapists.

I believe that you will be interested in the way in which I treat patients. It is no secret, and I will gladly describe the course of the treatment I give my patients. My patient sits on a chair, with his/her back parallel with the chair, hands on his/her thighs, palms facing the ceiling. If he or she is immobile, he/she can lie.

During the treatment, I do not touch the patient. I do not use the technique which involves touching, that is used by those with weak emission power.

I transmit energy mostly from the palms and fingertips, while I occasionally turn on the more powerful sources of emission: The third eye and solar plexus, but only in the situations when I deem it necessary to increase the emission power. I do this when I feel that the patient's organism is ready to withstand that much energy. While treating a patient, I am 100% focused, even if we are surrounded with people talking or loud music.

During the treatment session, I feel the energy flowing from my hands and in that way I discover (diagnose) the organism's problems. This way of diagnosing is absolutely reliable. The patients who have not previously revealed their problems to me or showed me the medical documentation regularly confirm my findings. I need not mention that I strictly follow the rules I have described (hands from down upwards). This is logical and natural, because that is the direction in which blood flows through the body. I return several times to the organs that give strong signals, sometimes chaotically absorbing bioenergy they need. When I feel that the energetic balance is restored, my intervention is over.

Therefore, my bioenergy and the organism of the patient are in constant contact, all the time until the end of the session. But, since bioenergy has extended effect, the cooperation doesn't end then. The energy that has "moved in" into an organism continues to work for 24 hours a day, for days after the treatment! I respect medications, but only Nature and natural ways of healing can accomplish something like that.

It is especially interesting, since it is totally unknown to the public, that during the treatment, a bioenergotherapist (including myself) transmits from his/her hands three kinds of energy: Heat, Electric and magnetic. We know that the organism is a unity and that the organs are interconnected, that every organ is important and necessary part of the whole. That is why I treat a patient from head to toes (literally). By that, I activate the complete organism of the patient and increase its defense mechanism, and no problem can escape my attention. After all, every part of the body is full of acupuncture points and centers and when they are all supplied with energy, there can be no mistake. The result has to be positive.

It is extremely important to point out another fact. I have already said that I transmit three kinds of energies during the treatment. Which one the organism is going to absorb, it depends only on the patient. His organism chooses according by its needs, it is not up to me! When the therapy is over, the organism that has received a bioenergetic "transfusion" determines the amount of energy and transports it to the causes of its problems. That is the perfection of nature at work.

Generally, I don't like discussing publicly the cases and conditions in which I have contributed to the healing, and I especially avoid mentioning the patients' names. Yet, since people like reading about that, I will describe some of the cases from my practice, protecting the privacy of patients as much as possible.

One of my "old" patients, and now my friend is an economy master V.P., owner and director of medications factory. Around ten years ago he had had a car crash. The consequence was a huge dark hematoma, stretching from his knee to the foot. This problem has caused strong pains and difficulties in walking, so he has come to me. After several treatments everything was OK, the hematoma was gone. After that, he has brought members of his family, pharmacists, and workers to me for treatment.

A couple of years after that V.P. has got an ABLATION of the eye cornea. He went to the ophthalmologist, a doctor with whom he was also a friend. She has examined him and told him that he needs an urgent surgery, in order to avoid blindness. He has thanked her for the advice, sat in his car and came to me. I have treated him for four consecutive days. After returning to his town, he went to his doctor again. After examining him, as he has later told me, she sighed and said: "Oh my, what have I been taught all these years?!" Of course, there was no sign of ablation.

Not long after that, V.P. has brought to me his worker, who has had an advanced tumor on her uterus. Besides, she was also pregnant. The doctors had advised the termination of pregnancy and tumor surgery. I don't remember exactly how many times she had come to me. What's important is the end result—the tumor had shrunk so much that she was able to give birth to a healthy child!

A dentist V.D., who has lived and worked in Germany for twenty years, has come to me in 1990. He brought with him his ten-year-old son who had an allergy of unknown cause. He has had suffocation seizures and often had a rash all over his body. His father had taken him to several physicians in Germany, but to no avail. After five treatments by me, the boy was healed, and his father had invited me to visit him.

During my stay in Bochum (Germany), my host has organized a dinner to which he had invited some of his dentist colleagues, and several prominent doctors from Dusseldorf, accompanied by their wives. When meeting them, I have noticed that one of the doctors' head is visibly shaking. Later, during dinner, he has tried to reach the bowl with salad on the table, but had given up, because his hands were shaking too much. He had noticed that I was watching him, so he just smiled sourly and drank a glass of whisky which was in front of him. His wife looked at him and said that the alcohol will destroy him. "His arms and head are shaking for twelve years, and yet he doesn't think about quitting alcohol", she added. When I remarked that drinking is not the cause of his problems, they have looked at me curiously. I have named his more than visible ossification of the neck part of the spine (spondylosis) as the source of the problem. They knew what I do and the doctor has asked me if bioenergy can help in any way. I have suggested that we go to one of the rooms, do a treatment, and he will have a chance to see the effects of bioenergy for himself. He rose from the table immediately, and we went to another room.

The guests have met our return with their eyes focused on the smiling doctor. He sat next to his wife, turned towards her and kissed her on the cheek. She has put her hand on his neck and said: "Oh, that thing on your neck has really shrunk!"

"Look at this!"—he stretched his arms up front—they were no longer shaking.

Then he stood up, approached me and started hugging me.

"Let my doctor live for two hundred years!" he exclaimed.

The other doctors and their wives have started asking me about the possibilities of solving their health problems. Soon after, some of them have had their first "meeting" with bioenergy.

It is interesting that three doctors have asked me whether bioenergy could help with the illnesses of some of their patients.

When I answered positively, they said that they will notify their patients tomorrow.

In later conversation, the doctors have suggested that I stay in Dusseldorf and work there, forever if I will, as one of them said.

For the next three weeks, I have treated patients in a house in Bochum, mainly those sent by the mentioned doctors, before I had to go back home.

Unfortunately, most of the doctors are still skeptical on the issue. Yet, whether they want it or not, the doctors and I do cooperate. A large number of doctors have come to me for treatment, but they have asked me not to tell anyone—so they wouldn't have problems with colleagues who do not appreciate bioenergy.

Once a gynecologist came to me asking whether he can send his patients to me, because he has seen that with several women I have treated, the therapy gave great results. Of course we have cooperated, and only he and I knew about it!

A wife of one of my acquaintances has great problems with her sight and goes to Moscow several times a year, where she receives special injections for expanding her eye capillaries. More out of curiosity, my acquaintance had asked me to do a couple of treatments of his wife. While we were sitting at the table in his apartment, his wife said that she sees better now. He just waived with his hand. She then told the time on the clock on the wall and recognized some smaller objects in the room, adding that she wasn't able to do that before. Her husband looked at her and me in disbelief. Soon after, she went to Russia again to receive her special injections. When she returned, she told about what happened to her in Moscow.

When she came to the clinic, Russian doctors have examined her. They were amazed and insisted that she tells them what she has done in the meantime since her last coming to Moscow, because they have determined that there has been a significant improvement of her vision. As they knew that was practically impossible, they have insisted that she reveals the kind of help she had been using. When she told them, they have asked her to help them come into contact with me, for the purpose of possible cooperation. That didn't happen, because it would mean that I would have to stay in Russia for a longer period, which I wasn't prepared to do.

It is known to the wider public that Russians, at some clinics, cooperate directly with bioenergotherapists. One of the most important ones is Juna (Dzuna). So, Russians know a lot about bioenergy and know that it can be used for scientific purposes, not only of medicinal nature.

Some ten years ago I was at Mallorca, Spain. There I have met Mr. H.E., owner of the tourist agency. His twenty-one-year-old daughter was suffering from scoliosis (side ossification and curving of the spine). When I saw her, I have diagnosed her problem. One shoulder was visibly lowered, also the head, and there was a clear mark of curving of the spine to the left on her back. Mr. H.E. tried to convince me that it happened because her breast have grown, although they were, if I may say, just a little bigger than mine! When he saw that he can't hide her problem, he had asked whether I could help. Five treatments were enough to straighten his daughter's spine and return in to a normal position.

On another occasion, also on Mallorca, I have met a certain Mr. Leonardo. During our first lunch together, he had complained that he often dreams about eating meat from the barbecue, but that he can only dream about it, because his doctor has determined that he was allergic to that food and forbade it. I was free to offer him my help.

"That is very kind of you, but I don't have much confidence in non-medicinal ways of treatment"—he said.

I didn't insist and it stayed at that. We continued to spend time together and once, while we were drinking coffee, he has asked me: "Did you mean it seriously when you said that you could help with my allergy?" When I answered affirmatively and guaranteed him that nothing bad could happen, quite the contrary, he agreed to the treatment.

After the therapy, I suggested that he order a portion of barbecue meat and eat it without fear. He hesitated, but still called the waiter.

When he ate the whole plate, he just looked at me timidly. Tomorrow he had called me on the phone and told me that I was a wizard. In the next few days we did four more treatments and the allergy was completely in the past.

The number of allergies is enormous. I have fought many of them, with success. It doesn't matter to me what the source of allergy is; I know what I should do and how to do it, the result always comes.

Here are some other examples from my practice:

Example 1: M.P. has spent his working years in a steel factory, from where he retired. He spent half of those years fighting Asthma. He has used the pump, without which he couldn't function. He came to me for help and we have done seven treatments. His condition improved after each treatment and at the end, the pump has ended on the shelf in his apartment as just a "memory of the bad days".

This was over fifteen years ago. I still see him sometimes and M.P. still breathes without using the pump.

Example 2: My cousin lives in a small village of some five hundred inhabitants, in which everybody knows everybody. Most of them are curious by nature and they know everything about one another.

My cousin's hip was attacked by coxarthrosis and she called me to come urgently, because she had great difficulties walking, she used a cane, while the villagers looked at her with pity, which irritated her even more.

I have gone there and in a couple of days, my cousin has walked from one end of the village to another, without the cane, to the amazement of the villagers.

Example 3: A young married couple had brought their three-year-old daughter to me. The child was stillborn and went blind while in the incubator. The parents have told me that the "number one" ophthalmologist in their town had tried to do something, but that he had given up quickly, saying that there is no chance that she will ever see. Every time I think about someone giving such a grim prognosis, it gives me the creeps. The chance for a cure, even if it is a minimal one, always exists, one should never give up. Therefore I recommend the doctors to speak for themselves and say "I can't do anything about it", instead of giving a definitive prognosis in the name of all possible ways of treatment!

I did a few treatments on the little girl, and she regained her sight. The parents then took her to the same ophthalmologist, who was shocked that the girl could see.

Example 4: The next example is that of a man whose voice cords were broken. That was said to me by his wife, adding that his speech comes down to hardly hearable and inarticulate whisper. In the hospital they were told that with long term treatment he could at best hope to restore 30% of his voice. I have accepted to treat him and after the second treatment he started talking again, not too loud, but articulate. After the fifth treatment his speech was restored completely.

About a week passed since then, when his wife called me on the phone again. She said that the previous day her husband was really yelling at the children, and that they were really scared. "It would be better if that man didn't help him"—their seven-year-old daughter told her mother.

Example 5: B.T., an owner of a workshop, was having troubles with leg and back pains. Also, one of his legs was swollen. Fifteen days of therapy in a famous institute at sea didn't help him either. Then his friend Z.L., a football player of one of the Belgrade clubs, recommended him to come to me for help. After the first therapy, he felt much better, while after the second therapy, the pain was gone. Even the leg stopped swelling.

Example 6: After an injury to the ligaments at the tournament in Australia, the doctor have recommended Z.L., a football player, to put on a leg cast, or even to have a surgery, which would've kept him away from the football field for at least three months. They brought him to me by carrying him, while he went home on foot! Twenty days later, he had started the preparations for the spring part of the championship.

Example 7: M.T. was present when I treated her nephew. I have noticed that she had a very swollen leg and I have suggested that I treat her as well. "I thought you were joking, since I have had that swelling for fifteen years. It is a result of a blow and on that spot the veins have dilated and the capillaries have burst. I could never wear boots because of it."—M.T. said.

After the first therapy, the swelling shrank, skin loosened, while the red color of the capillaries started to fade. After two more treatments, the trouble she had had for years was history. Improvement was more than visible, her colleagues at work have also noticed it.

Example 8: A family from Belgrade had a car crash. Their six and a half-year-old child had the worst injuries—open fracture of the foot. The boy was treated in a hospital, but the wound didn't heal even after a month.

"I have confidence in bioenergy, so I have brought the boy to you"—his mother, a technology engineer, said. When I saw the wound, I told her that one treatment will be enough and that it will heal. I have also told her that the doctor's examination would confirm it. That's exactly what happened. Right after the first treatment, the boy started walking, and his walk improved with every next day.

Example 9: The next example is Z.V. who was suffering from intolerable pain because of the stone in his kidney. His friends wanted to help him and they recommended me. After the first treatment, the pains were gone. Here is the story in his words:

"It is true, I must admit, that Bralic helped me, although I was always against bioenergy and alternative medicine. I was in terrible pains, I crawled on the floor, hit my head against the wall. In 28 hours I have had seven one hour seizures. After the first session, I felt relief. While my therapist and my friends were drinking coffee, I fell asleep. When I woke up, I felt like I was born again. The pains were completely gone!"

Example 10: Mrs. M.P. was troubled by fatigue, dizziness, pain in the arms. She couldn't even sit on a chair with a hard seat. She went to the doctor and an ultrasound found a tumor on her uterus. After five or six bioenergetic treatments, her problems were gone, and an ultrasound showed that the tumor had disappeared.

Example 11: A young woman, J.K. has come to me because of visibly enlarged and cystic Thyroid Gland, which was threatening to turn into Basedow's disease. Her physician had suggested a surgery and she was very upset because of it.

After the fifth treatment I have suggested that she visits her physician and check the condition of her problem. The results were positive: Thyroid Gland was back to normal, the cysts were gone, so the surgery plan was cancelled.

Regarding this example, I would like to point out that the problem with thyroid gland was mostly reserved for women for decades. In the last years, this rule no longer applies; the number of men facing this illness grows daily, it has almost reached the number of women with this problem. Unfortunately, even the children aren't spared.

Example 12: Here's an interesting case. While visiting a friend, I have met his neighbor who dropped by with her six-month-old baby in a stroller. As a consequence of a complicated delivery, the child was left with one foot turned more to the inside. The prognoses were not encouraging. Young woman has asked me whether bioenergy can do something to help her baby. I said that I hope so, and did a short treatment of a baby, that was sleeping in the stroller.

My hope came true and the baby's foot soon went back to normal.

Example 13. There hardly is a man, especially after 40, who has been spared the problems with Prostate. Getting up five or six times at night to go to the toilet is certainly unpleasant. As I have treated a large number of men with this problem, I can only say that, regardless of their age, there was an improvement with every one of them, while most of them got rid of the problem with prostate for a longer period.

Example 14: Sinusitis is a usually a chronic disease followed by strong pains in the front part of the head (behind the forehead). It was also the case with L.L., to whom I have done five treatments. Almost a month after that, L.L. has every day, as he said, filled five or six towels with pus that came out of his nose. How can that much pus be inside a man's head, as a consequence of an inflammation that has lasted for years, is difficult to explain.

Example 15: A mole is an almost inevitable "decoration" on a human body. It is not dangerous, but if it gets irritated by scratching, a blow or any kind of injury, it can become very dangerous. "It is a cancer at the doorstep"—said one doctor, with whom I fully agree. An injury to the mole on the back has brought to me a middle-aged man. His mole looked as if it was cut with a knife, with traces of fresh bleeding and redness. A man said that he has been putting compresses on it, but to no avail, and that his doctor had advised him to have a surgery. I have done a treatment on him. The day after, he called me on the phone. "When I woke up this morning, as usual, I touched my back. As I couldn't feel the mole, I have called my wife to have a look and tell me what has happened to it. On the spot where the mole was, stood only a trace of slightly lighter skin. In the bed I have later found a crust that had been created on the mole during the night, which had later dried up and fell off."

Even I didn't expect this serious problem to be solved so quickly, so I was also very pleasantly surprised.

Example 16: I have gladly accepted the invitation by two friends to visit them in the editorial office of their magazine. At the arranged time, when entering the office, I saw an unusually large number of people, who were visibly upset. Someone yelled: "Call an ambulance!" I have seen the technical editor who told me the chief editor's back had stiffened and he was lying helplessly on the table.

I have asked them to turn him to the side and hold him in that position for ten minutes. I advised them not to call an ambulance and started treating this unplanned patient. Fifteen minutes later, the editor got up and said: "Now, everyone back to work!" He thanked me and went to his office.

Example 17: The aforementioned forty-year-old V.P. came to me and asked me to help him with the consequences of a car crash he had three years ago. There was still a visible hematoma on his knee, while his leg under the knee was full of scars and hematomas. But it was his strabismus that has attracted my attention. The iris of his eye was almost in the corner of his eye when he was looking straight in front of him. An ophthalmologist had told him that it couldn't be helped, because he had been born with that problem.

We have conducted seven treatments. Everything went well with the leg, while the iris returned nearly all the way to the center of the eye. The ophthalmologist was surprised with the 70% improvement of strabismus and happy that he was wrong with the prognosis.

Many people who do or have treated others with bioenergy, I know for sure, have accepted only the patients with milder health problems. That's why they have achieved some progress in the treatment.

Unlike them, a real challenge for me have always been the diseases and conditions considered difficult, especially those that are supposedly incurable. My creed is: if you don't try, you'll never know whether you could do something.

There is almost no illness that I haven't fought with and, fortunately, I was successful even then when no one thought it was possible. That way, I came to the conclusions about the causes of some difficult illnesses, but I would rather talk about it on another occasion. My findings are justified in a simple way—in practice: if I have found the source of a certain illness, I treat all the patients in the same way, by energetically "attacking" the source of the problem, and if there is always a positive result, it is clear that I have discovered the source. When you know the source of the problem, it is easier to solve it.

Americans have published the information that the most common causes of death are Heart Disease, Cancer and Medical Errors.

I have named this data not with the intention of accusing the doctors; every man can make a mistake, and doctors are also human.

I feel obliged to tell you that, when I treat a patient with bioenergy, there is not the slightest chance that I could hurt him! Before I have fully devoted myself to treating people with bioenergy, I have systematically checked whether there could be a danger for the patient due to my intervention. I have tested members of my family and several friends, whose consent I have received. When I was 100% sure that there is no danger for my patients, I have devoted myself to being a bioenergotherapist.

Organic Diseases Cause Psychic Diseases

18

The tempo of life is getting faster, economic crisis has spread around the world, unemployment is rising, and the people are exposed to constant stress. That contributes to an alarming increase of the number of people suffering from health problems of psychic nature.

Until a few years ago I didn't commit to working on psychic diseases. One of the reasons for that was the fact that people with these problems rarely came to me for help, probably rejecting the possibility that bioenergy could help.

Since the moment when a famous psychiatrist told me in confidence that medicine cannot do much about psychic problems, I was intrigued and decided to commit myself more to this problem.

Almost everyone has heard the saying that "all the problems come from the head". By helping people with psychic problems I have come to a conclusion that this is not entirely true. My experience allows me to say that in more than 30% of cases organic problems cause psychic problems! With most patients I would at start determine the problems with the neck part of the spine (spondylosis), which decreases the inflow of blood into the head. There were also problems with the thyroid gland and the stomach, which is the most sensitive organ. Almost every time, when I succeed in solving the problems of these organs, psychic condition of the patient would be significantly improved.

Here is an example from my practice that confirms my thesis about the influence of organic problems on psychic problems.

An acquaintance has called me on the phone a while ago. He said that his fifteen-year-old son had been placed into "Children's psychiatry". He added that his son did have problems lately, especially with occasional feeling of fear, but that he was unpleasantly surprised with his placing onto psychiatry. Of course, he had asked if I could help his son.

Tomorrow we went together into a visit to his son. We found him sitting on one of the four beds, alone in a room with bars on the windows. Immediately after entering that depressive room, I have sensed an unpleasant, negative energetic charge. "How does the boy feel?"—I wondered.

He stood up to greet us. I have immediately noticed the ossification at the neck part of his spine, which visibly limited the movements of his head to the sides and caused his shoulders to be leaned forward. His problems with the thyroid gland were also apparent. As soon as I have put my hand on his neck, the middle-aged woman, clinical psychiatrist entered the room.

She stared at me and asked: "Who are you?" In a moment I managed to tell a lie—that I was her colleague, a psychiatrist and a relative of the boy. "And why are you touching his neck?"—she continued to question me.

"I feel that his spine is not in order, also the thyroid gland and the stomach"—I had decided to "test" her.

"Even if it were so, what would that have to do with his psychic problems?"—she had asked me disparagingly.

"My dear colleague, I think that the organism is a whole and that all organs can help each other out, as well as disturb one another"—I replied.

"Is that logical? Anyway, that's an interesting point of view"—she said and left the room.

While I was treating the boy, his father was standing "guard" at the door, so that no one would come in. As soon as we have finished, his mood had visibly improved and he said that he felt much better. I have suggested that he straightens his shoulders, and that's exactly what he did, turning his head left-right, up-down with ease. Also, we could hear his stomach growling, with occasional belching, because this organ was until then "blocked". The thyroid gland had also received its "medicine", his neck had "thinned" and he said that he doesn't have problems swallowing anymore (which usually accompanies the problem with the thyroid gland). I have reminded him that we ought to repeat the treatment a couple more times and we have left him with a smile on his face.

His father and I came to visit him the day after. After the treatment the boy had told us that he had started to walk more often in the park of the clinic (they were allowed to do so), to read a book, magazines, talk to other patients, sleep well, and that the previously felt fears were replaced by the feeling of self-confidence!

Three days later we have visited him again and repeated the treatment.

This time he told us that the psychiatrist with whom we have spoken during our first visit had started to send him to spine exercises, and that she has also looked at his neck.

We have visited him two-three times more and the boy was soon released from this institution as cured. Since then, he has no health problems, psychic or organic.

Parkinson's Disease

19

During my bioenergotherapeutic practice I have come into contact with people suffering from Parkinson's disease, multiple sclerosis, epilepsy, stroke, brain tumor....

Even before they came to me, I knew that they must surely suffer from significant ossification of the neck which causes the decrease of inflow of blood into the head and, in time, contributes to appearance of these illnesses. It is also followed by reduction of the gray brain mass and motor system disorders.

I have come to a basic conclusion that it is the ossification and the blockade of the inflow of blood into the head that is the main reason of these illnesses and conditions. Since bioenergy is efficient in removing the named problems, I have had significant success in treating these illnesses.

I would especially like to say something about Parkinson's disease. The number of people suffering from it around the world is worrying. For example, almost half of the inhabitants of New York have problems with some form of Parkinson's!

It is a very complex disease that causes dramatic motor system disorder, lack of gray brain mass, often complete immobility, limited ability of speech, uncontrollable shaking of hands (tremor) and practically cuts the patient out of the normal course of life. Treatment of this disease is permanent—by medications for life, at least for now. Yet, I must point out that I have successfully cured one patient from Parkinson's disease completely, and, to amazement of his colleagues, who have already predicted him an early retirement, brought him back to work!

But, there is a big, almost unsolvable problem. Patients suffering from Parkinson's disease take medications several times a day, in such quantities that their positive effects are almost minimal when compared with the negative effects. A well-known physician, specialist in this field, has told me once that the medications have a positive effect on the patient for approximately half an hour, while the other couple of hours, until taking new doses, have negative effects on the organism!

That fact has created me great trouble, because I was forced to fight against two powerful opponents—the disease and negative effects of strong medications. Therefore, I have stopped treating patients suffering from Parkinson's disease on a regular basis.

On the one hand, I do not want to meddle into the work of physicians and take responsibility by advising patients to stop taking medications, which is hardly feasible because their organisms have already developed dependency on the medications. On the other hand, this double fight slows the effects of bioenergy, so I have decided to dedicate myself to fighting other illnesses, whose number is, unfortunately, great.

Many of you know that treating drug dependency is performed by gradual decrease of the doses of drugs the patient takes. Logically, a sudden stop of taking drugs would cause grave consequences in the organism of someone who is drug-dependent for years. It is similar with medications, not so much as with drug addicts, but the addiction of the organism is already present with a great number of people on medications, especially with difficult illnesses. Parkinson's disease is one of them. Apart from that, the treatment of drug addiction is performed in special clinics, in which time is not of great importance, while I can't allow myself that "luxury", because there is a great number of people that need my help, whose problems I can solve relatively quickly and successfully.

I sincerely hope that it is just a matter of time when medicine will find a cure for Parkinson's disease.

Brain is the "commander in chief" of the organism. Inside the brain is an invaluable gland—Pineal Gland. Medicine knows about its existence, it is shown on the head CT, but we know almost nothing about it! When the doctors open up the skull, in touch with oxygen, the pineal gland simply disappears.

I admit I know nothing about that gland and the way it functions, but I do know that bioenergy has positive effects on it and its activity, because bioenergy doesn't need to open the skull, it enters every organ quickly and easily, without the danger of causing any problems.

Bioenergy is a gift of nature to humankind, I believe you will agree.

Recipes for Healing Potions, Compresses, Balms, Self-help

20

Recipe 1: For the improvement of Circulation, Digestion, helps Ejection of Toxins from the organism, Clears the Lungs, helps with Hemorrhoids

Take a 2 dl cup and put three teaspoons of honey into it, pour boiled water to fill half of the cup and mix. Add two teaspoons of apple vinegar, one teaspoon of minced cinnamon and 5-6 drops of oil (preferably olive oil). Add hot water to fill the cup, mix and drink on an empty stomach.

Recipe 2: Diabetes

Minced nuts, apple vinegar and yoghurt are used for this recipe. Let your measure be a coffee cup, while you should keep the potion in a small jar. Pour the minced nuts, apple vinegar and yoghurt into a jar, mix it and keep it refrigerated. Every morning take one teaspoon of the potion on an empty stomach, which you should mix first every time.

This potion lowers elevated blood sugar.

Recipe 3: Gastritis, Stomach Ulcer

Stomach is the most sensitive organ and almost everyone has sometimes had problems with it. This recipe will help you, especially if you suffer from gastritis or stomach ulcer. At least once a day, on an empty stomach, have a few bites of fresh cabbage leaf, and then don't eat for an hour after it. This vegetable will be your personal physician.

Recipe 4: Liver

Liver is a very important organ, while its problems are more than dangerous. I must point out that I have been a witness of the healing of several people suffering from Hepatitis C and several from Liver Cirrhosis.

Like the previous recipe with cabbage, also on an empty stomach, two or three times a day, chew Trappist Cheese. It is a perfect cleaner of the liver.

Recipe 5: Paradentosis

One of the proven ways to at least slow down the receding of the gums, in many cases make the gums return to previous condition is this: take one tablespoon of olive, pumpkin or sunflower oil, gargle it for twenty minutes. Don't swallow it, but hold it in your mouth and occasionally gargle. After twenty minutes spit it out. It is recommended that you do it every day. The oil helps your gums, but also draws the toxins out from your organism.

Recipe 6: Increasing the Activity of Your Bioenergy

This recipe is also simple. Mince a tablespoon of dry figs, a tablespoon of dry plums and a tablespoon of dry grapes; put it into a bowl with water so that the mass is completely under the surface. In the morning, eat the prepared mass on an empty stomach. It will be an energetic bomb for your organism, in a positive sense, clearly. Repeat this two or three times a month, which is quite enough.

Recipe 7: A Boil (Under the Skin or on it)

A person could hardly be found that hasn't had problems with boils. It can appear on various places on the body.

Mix the same quantities of honey and flour in a cup. Put the mixture on the place where the boil has appeared and cover with a bandage. Hold it for a few hours and if the mixture hasn't driven the pus to the surface, put a new mixture.

Recipe 8: Breast Problems

Statistics has registered a sudden increase in number of breast cancer patients in the world. One of the causes for this disease is wearing bras made from synthetic materials and carrying plastic pencils in pockets on the chest. This may sound funny, but it has been scientifically proven.

You can move your pencil into your briefcase or a purse, while the bras should always be made from natural materials. Plastic and synthetic materials, when in direct contact with the body, pose a danger for health.

Compresses

As I am a big fan of sports, I would like to give some advice to athletes and amateurs on how to heal their injuries faster and return to training.

1. Potato Compress

A potato is cooked without removing the crust, mashed, put onto a bandage and, while still warm, put onto the spot where the blow had been received.

2. Cabbage Compress

Pour hot water onto a cabbage leaf and put it onto the place of the concussion or swelling.

3. Onion Compress

Clean and cut two or three onion head into pieces, put it on a napkin then put it onto the injured place and wrap with nylon. Finally, wrap everything with a woolen scarf.

The choice of the compress is up to you.

Self-help

1. One of the ways for self-help is auto stimulation of the acupuncture points on the ears, by which you can strengthen the defense mechanism of your organism.

Use your thumbs and forefingers to press the lower, soft part of your ears. Press it harder, until it hurts very much. Do not weaken the grip for ten seconds. Then move your fingers to the edge of the ears, also to the soft part, and repeat the pressing routine. Repeat this gradually moving the pressure towards the top of the ears. During this exercise, you will feel warmth, which is a sign that you have activated a great number of acupuncture points in your body. After you have pressed the top of your ears, the exercise is over.

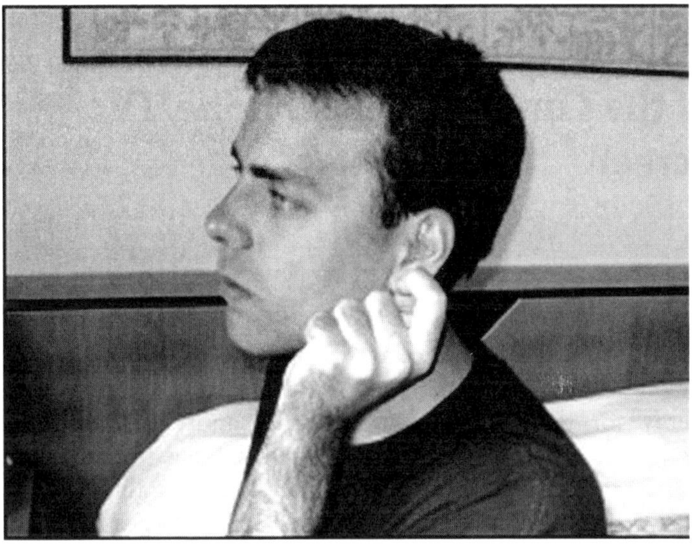

Do not exercise longer than two or three minutes.

2. If you have problems with your sinuses (paranasal), I advise you to occasionally chew honeycomb.

3. For strengthening hair roots and to prevent dandruff, I advise putting diluted lemon juice on your hair after washing it, while it is still wet. After a couple of minutes, wash it out of your hair.

4. Cod liver oil is efficient in removing dots and skin stains from the skin, most frequently from the arms. It is also good in removing scars, regardless how old they are.

Take a small piece of cotton wool, dip it into cod liver oil and rub the skin for two-three minutes. After a short break you can repeat it. Do it two or three times a day.

By applying small quantities of cod liver oil on your eyelashes, you will increase their volume.

How to Neutralise the Radiation of the Computer, Cell Phone, TV Screen

21

There hardly is a home today without a computer or TV, or a person without a cell phone. As electricity is the provider of energy for these devices, a certain quantity of radiation is inevitable. Whether the radiation is damaging for our health, and to what extent, is another matter. Is it desirable to protect oneself from excessive exposure to radiation, just in case? I think—of course. Therefore, some advice follow.

Computer

I must agree with those opinions that classify excessive use of this machine as an addiction. Let's see what we can do to minimize our exposure to its emission.

1. Draw the keyboard nearer to you, to increase your distance from the screen.
2. While working, turn your body at least a little to the side, instead of directly towards the screen, to avoid direct exposure to radiation.
3. Occasionally move away from the computer for a couple of minutes. When you go to the bathroom, use the opportunity to wash your hands with cold water. That way you will get rid of at least a part of accumulated radiation.

Advice 1. and 2. also apply to watching TV.

Cell Phone

Don't keep it in a shirt pocket, inner jacket pocket, near the stomach or the liver.

One doctor had told me about some girl who had troubles with her stomach. When she arrived, he had noticed that she carries her cell phone around her neck and that it lies exactly on her stomach. He had advised her to move it into her purse and after a few days her problems with the stomach were gone. Therefore, you have briefcases, hand purses, purses, etc. at your disposal; if you carry it in them, your cell phone will not endanger your health. Spare yourself the unnecessary risk.

The following example may create an impression that I am against technic, but that isn't so. I regard technic as a need of the modern age, something that helps people to function with more ease in the fast tempo of everyday life.

A couple of years ago, two Russian journalists have placed an egg on the table. Then one of them put his cell phone on the table, facing the egg, about 10 cm away. His colleague did the same thing. After fifteen minutes, the egg was warm. After half an hour, the egg was hard boiled!

The Bushmen are a very hospitable people. When meeting strangers, they are prepared to share all their modest possessions. Their smiles radiate positive energy. But, if you wish to take a photo or film them with a camera, they will ask you not to do so. They believe that cameras take away their energy?! It's hard to tell whether that's true, but that is what they feel by intuition.

Healing By Your Own Bioenergy—Practical Application

22

We have already said that every human being possesses bioenergy, but little is known about the way it can be activated to help the preservation of health. It can be used as preventive and as a medicine for many illnesses. Hence the advice about the ways you can activate your bioenergy are sure to attract your attention.

Increasing pollution, air humidity and climate changes have contributed to exposure of respiratory organs to bronchitis, asthma, pneumonia.... With a little patience and a little persistence, you are determined to heal yourself. Follow this advice: sit, put your hands on your knees with your fingers stretched, while your palms are facing upwards. Stay in that position for 5-6 minutes. Then put your hands on your chest if you have problems with bronchitis or on your lungs if you have a cold, pneumonia or asthma. Hold your hands on that place for ten minutes. You will feel the inflow of heat energy into your chest, which will alleviate breathing. Inhale deeply and check whether that has already happened. Then lower your arms next to your body, shake them strongly a couple of times and then put them back on your knees, with the palms facing upwards. Repeat the routine two or three times. When you decide to finish this kind of auto-therapy, inhale deeply several times and you will certainly have the impression that more air gets into your lungs. Wash your hands with cold water, then get back to your activities, while bioenergy continues to work for your organism.

This kind of treatment is also efficient against all kinds of allergies.

Women can treat their problems with the ovaries, and also men with prostate, in the following way: sit comfortably on a couch or an armchair, put your hands on your knees with palms facing upwards for a few minutes. Then put your hands on the place where your ovaries or your prostate is and your heat energy will flow into these organs, performing its therapeutic role.

If you are suffering from problems with your heart, it is desirable that you put your hand, which you have previously held briefly facing upwards, to the middle of your chest, making 7-8 circular movements. That is self-massage with your own bioenergy, which improves the activity of the heart and prevents arrhythmia.

Digestion can be improved in just a few minutes: put your fingertips (excluding the thumbs) on your stomach. Press harder and move lower, also pressing, all the way to the lower stomach. It is certain that you will occasionally hear your bowels working, which will be the sign that the digestion has improved. Do the same routine in the area of your Liver and Pancreas, in order to improve their work.

Varicose Veins, Leg and Feet Cramps, Celulitis are the consequence of bad circulation. One of the ways to tackle this problem is this: put your hands on one thigh, one hand on the inner side, the other on the outer side. By gently and briefly pressing, go down with your hands all the way to the foot. Then put your hands back into the starting position and repeat the routine several times. Do the same with the other leg.

Make sure that you move your hands downwards, and not the other way, because that would be contrary to the natural blood flow.

Problems with the thyroid gland are ever more present, even at young children. Bioenergy is a formidable opponent to this enemy of the health.

During the day, occasionally touch the back of your neck and move your hands to the throat, on both sides, with quick movements. This helps the thyroid gland, as well as the blood flow in the carotid artery.

Rheumatic problems usually appear in arm wrists, ankle joints, shoulders and knees. Bioenergy is efficient against these problems as well. People suffering from rheumatic problems often make themselves warm, which sometimes eases their problems. So, heat energy is crucial in facing this unpleasant and painful problem. But, that doesn't mean that any source of heat can solve the problem. If you stand by the radiator, the heat will feel good. But, when you step away from it, your organism immediately stops receiving heat. That's not the case with bioenergy—it enters the organism and stays there for days, sometimes months.

Your bioenergy is the source of magnetic, electric and heat energy, which means that you will be able to help yourself with rheumatic problems, too.

Your hands are in this case also your therapist.

Putting the palms of your hands on the places suffering from rheumatic problems is a reliable way of healing yourself.

Of course, it is necessary to charge yourself with Cosmic Energy by holding your hands with the palms facing upwards.

During life, a person functions best when his/her health condition is stable, physically and psychically. But, everyone has sometimes faced an illness, whether more or less dangerous.

Medicine is there to help, but why wouldn't you do something for yourself, for preserving your health and, if necessary, helping your organism defeat an illness?

If you can't fully succeed yourself, you will at least help those that you seek help from.

Being passive, on any issue, is not helpful. Relying only on the help of others, when health is already impaired, is not a good attitude.

By using advice from this book, you are given an opportunity to keep your immune system on the level required to protect you from health problems. You are also given an opportunity to defeat some of the illnesses that may have already attacked your organism. These advice have helped many people, so why wouldn't they help you, too?

Index